Nursing Process Manual:

Assessment Tool for the
Roy Adaptation Model

Joan M. Seo-Cho, R.N., M.N.

Assistant Professor of Nursing
Mount St. Mary's College, Los Angeles, CA

Polaris Publishing

Glendale, California

Assessment Tool for the Roy Adaptation Model

Copyright © 1999, Joan M. Seo-Cho

ISBN: 0-9669791-0-9

First Printing, January 1999
Second Printing, June 1999
Third Printing, January 2000
Fourth Printing, September 2000
Fifth Printing, September 2001
Sixth Printing, September 2002

Published by Polaris Publishing
P.O. Box 11252
Glendale, CA 91226 USA
Fax: (626) 576-7727

Printed in Canada

Table of Contents

Foreword

This assessment tool for the Roy Adaptation Model is an important contribution to the literature that helps to bridge the gap between theory and practice. The Roy Adaptation Model has been in use for nearly 30 years and a significant number of publications are available. Assessment parameters are integrated into basic texts on the model and assessment guides for given clinical situations appear occasionally in nursing journals. However, no one publication provides a complete and up-to-date discussion of the nursing process and a guide for nursing assessment based on all four adaptive modes of the model. Joan Seo-Cho has filled this gap by presenting a complete assessment tool for the Roy Adaptation Model in the format of a nursing process manual.

Ms. Cho is highly qualified to present this manual since she has developed and refined the assessment content while teaching the model for nearly 25 years at Mount St. Mary's College in Los Angeles, where the model was initially developed. She is my colleague and friend, who over these years has authored several chapters in the basic texts on the model. Ms. Cho has generously shared her work with students and with other faculty who have found the assessment tool to be most helpful in understanding the model and applying it to clinical practice.

It is time to make this important work available to a wider audience. I am indeed grateful that Ms. Cho has been able to publish this work for students, faculty, and practicing nurses. The assessment tool provides a useful resource to anyone who seeks to link the use of the Roy Model with nursing practice.

Sister Callista Roy, R.N., Ph.D., FAAN
Professor and Nurse Theorist
School of Nursing, Boston College,
Chestnut Hill, Massachusetts

Introduction

The primary purpose of developing this manual was in providing the beginning level Adaptation Nursing students with a practical guide for how to proceed with nursing process according to the Roy Adaptation Model of Nursing. It is to be used as a companion clinical handbook for the main text of the Roy Adaptation Model Nursing.

The Roy Model considers the recipients of nursing care to include collectives such as families, groups, organizations, communities, and society as a whole, as well as human beings as individuals. The advanced level students will, eventually, be involved in the care of all or some of those collectives and be able to carry out the nursing processes to promote adaptation in those collectives. However, it is the beginning level students who will have the most difficulty in conceptualizing and implementing the major components of the model in a practical manner in clinical situations. Therefore, it is this author's intention to provide the very beginning level students with a practical tool to learn how to proceed with the nursing process according to the Roy Adaptation Model, in an adult individual care setting.

Carrying out the nursing process according to the tool will provide an excellent opportunity to exercise the student's critical thinking process. For each adaptive mode, the interrelationships among the six (6) steps of the nursing process are to be clearly understood.

Each adaptive mode is presented with:

1. An introduction to the particular need/mode to set the major focus, which lists possible nursing diagnoses and the manifesting cluster of behaviors for each diagnosis.

2. A list of specific behaviors that are to be assessed to check out the person's current adaptation status in the particular need/mode, and the norms for the behaviors for a comparison with actual behaviors assessed.

3. A list of particular groups of stimuli that are considered to be the major stimuli (influencing factors) for the particular need/mode

in order to identify which particular stimuli or stimulus has caused the ineffective behaviors/adaptation problem(s) in the need/mode.

4. A list of possible nursing diagnosis/adaptation problems that can be identified on the basis of assessment using the tool.

Also included in the manual is a special section, as a convenient reference, of an overview of psychosocial developmental tasks for each stage of the human person's life. The developmental tasks are considered to be the sociocultural norms of the society. The society expects and mostly accepts them as norm. Therefore, the developmental tasks are to be used as criteria for judgment in assessment of adaptation in the psychosocial modes. It is important for the student to be familiar with what is usually expected of the person in that particular stage of life before attempting to assess the individual's actual adaptation in the psychosocial modes.

The Purpose of Nursing Assessment
A Philosophical Statement

The purpose of Nursing Assessment according to the Basic Needs approach of the Adaptation Model is not in identifying the client's medical problem. Though nursing does participate in the process, diagnosis and treatment of disruptions in the client's body structure and function are ultimately the role function of the medical profession. The purpose of nursing assessment is to identify the client's adaptation problem in order to plan and implement interventions which do not necessarily need a physician's collaboration.

It is evident that both the nursing and medical assessment include many of the same behaviors. However, each assessment has its own unique primary purpose: Medicine focuses on the identification of the type and extent of the disruption in the structure and function, while nursing focuses on the person's responses to the disruption. In other words, medical assessment is primarily concerned with finding out, as accurately as possible, what body parts and functions are damaged and to what extent. In comparison, nursing assessment deals with how the person's ability to meet daily basic needs is affected by the damage and other circumstantial stimuli. Therefore, nursing assessment, especially at a beginning level, does not need to have a long exhaustive list of behaviors to be assessed, as medical assessment does. One should not confuse nursing assessment with medical assessment which uses the body systems approach.

There are certain behaviors that are representative of the person's status as to whether the person's particular basic needs are adequately or insufficiently met at a given time. These are the behaviors the nurse will independently assess and simply monitor to see whether the needs are adequately or inadequately met. Only these behaviors related to the basic needs are listed in the enclosed tool. And, **the problems to be diagnosed through the nursing assessment are the adaptation problems in maintaining, regaining, or promoting one's health to the best of one's capability in a given situation.**

In summary, the following example can be used to clarify the different but overlapping nature of nursing assessment: When an accident victim is admitted to the unit, **the physician will focus her/his assessment on the type and extent of the damage to the body structure and function, and the nurse will initially assist the physician in carrying out that task. However, the nurse will also begin her/his independent assessment to deal with the person's total responses to the situation and how the accident has and will affect the person's life through the four modes of Adaptation.** In this case, the structural and functional damages caused by the accident will be assessed as the major stimuli for the person's adaptation problem. The problem can manifest cross in different needs and modes. The accident may, initially, cause adaptation problems in the person's Rest and Activity need because of the medical restriction on the person's physical activity. However, the problem in the Rest and Activity need in turn may impose potential adaptation problems in other needs and modes; problems in Bowel Elimination and Protection needs, feeling of loss of physical control in Self Concept mode, and the challenges of occupying Sick Role are some examples. Having assessed these potential or actual adaptation problems, the nurse can intervene to assist the person in preventing or dealing effectively with the problems in order to promote healthy adaptation.

The Nursing Process

Patient's Initial: _____ Rm #: _____

Student's Name: _____

Primary Role: _____

Secondary Roles: _____

Maturation Stage: _____

Tertiary Roles: _____

Developmental Tasks: _____

1st Level Assessment: Assessment of Behaviors	2nd Level Assessment: Assessment of Stimuli	Nursing Diagnosis (3 components):	Nursing Goal:	Evaluation:
Assess all the behaviors according to the specific basic need and identify the ineffective behaviors by circling them.	Investigate all of the influencing factors listed in the tool and identify the negative stimuli by circling them.	Reviewing the ineffective behavior in the 1st level assessment: (1) Make a statement of the nursing problem the client is experiencing; (2) List the ineffective behaviors manifested for the specific problem; (3) List the causative stimuli according to the Focal, Contextual, and Residual Stimuli.	Looking at the diagnosis, state the client's nursing goal in terms of the client's behavioral outcome expected as the result of your nursing intervention, with an appropriate time frame. **Nursing Intervention:** List the nursing actions you are planning to carry out to assist the client/patient to achieve the goal stated above.	State as to whether the client's nursing goal is met or not; list the behaviors validating the outcome.

1) **Dx:**	Nursing Goal:
2) **Manifested by:** Ineffective behaviors a) b) c) 3) **Due to:** Stimuli affecting the behaviors Focal - Contextual - Residual -	Nursing Intervention:

SIX STEPS OF THE NURSING PROCESS
The Nursing Process: Roy Adaptation Model Approach

According to the Adaptation Model, there are six interrelated sequential (horizontal) steps to the Nursing Process:

1. **Assessment of Behaviors** – the 1st level assessment.

2. **Assessment of Stimuli** – the 2nd level assessment.

3. **Nursing Diagnosis** – identification of the adaptation problem.

4. **Goal Setting** – defining behavioral outcome to be achieved as result of nursing interventions.

5. **Planning/Implementing of Interventions** – formulating and executing the nursing actions to be carried out to assist the person to achieve the nursing goal.

6. **Evaluation/Modification** – assessing to see whether the goal is met or not met and to make change in action if necessary.

The First Step
Assessment of Behaviors: 1st Level Assessment

This step of the process involves assessment of the representative behaviors indicative of whether the person's particular Basic Need is adequately met or not met. When some of the behaviors are not within the norm, the behaviors are considered to be ineffective, meaning that the person's particular need is not adequately met and the individual is experiencing adaptation problem(s) at this time. The behaviors to be assessed are listed in the assessment tool. These behaviors are assessed by observations, interviewing, physical examination, measurement of the person's response to various stimuli.

In performing the 1st level assessment, the student learns:

1. *What* to assess: A particular set of behaviors which is representative of the adaptation status for each basic need or mode of adap-

tation, distinguishing the ineffective behaviors from the adaptive behaviors.

2. *Why* to assess: Significance of each behavior to be assessed for the particular basic need or mode of adaptation.

3. *How* to assess: Correct means of assessing each behavior.

The ultimate purpose of the 1st level assessment is to collect adequate data in order to make a judgment about the person's adaptation status in the particular need or mode. Once the data is collected, the behaviors are to be analyzed to identify each cluster of behaviors indicating a particular nursing diagnosis.

The Second Step
Assessment of Stimuli: 2nd Level Assessment

In Adaptation Nursing, a person is viewed as an adaptive system. And the behaviors (output) observed in the 1st level assessment are responses to certain stimuli (input). **The stimuli that promote Adaptive Responses (normal behaviors) are considered to be Positive stimuli, while stimuli that cause Ineffective Responses (abnormal behaviors) are considered to be Negative stimuli.**

In Adaptation Nursing, intervention is done by managing the impinging stimuli. Therefore, it becomes important to investigate the stimuli that cause ineffective responses in order to plan appropriate nursing interventions. An accurate identification of the causative stimuli sets the direction for setting realistic nursing goals and planning effective nursing intervention.

Assessment of stimuli is done by reviewing the major influencing factors listed in the tool for each particular basic need and mode. There are certain influential factors which are unique to each basic need/mode, and by reviewing each of those factors, one can identify the specific stimuli that cause the manifesting ineffective behaviors. These stimuli are not limited to the person's physiological, mental and emotional factors which affect the parson's adaptation status. The list also includes any environmental factors which are physical, socio-economical, political, or cultural in nature, whenever they are appropriate.

The assessment of stimuli is also helpful in identifying the potential adaptation problems which are not indicated at present, but may be forthcoming unless appropriate preventive nursing interventions are carried out in advance. For example, even though the 1st level assessment reveals no ineffective behaviors indicating nutritional problems at present time, the 2nd level assessment may reveal structural or functional disruptions in the person's gastrointestinal system which may interfere with the person's ingestion or absorption process. In this case, a nursing diagnosis of "Potential for a condition of malnutrition" could be derived. Therefore, all of the major influencing factors (as indicated in the process form) should be reviewed even if the 1st level assessment does not indicate an adaptation problem at the present time.

In performing the 2nd level assessment, the student learns to determine:

1. The major influencing factors that impact one's ability to meet each particular basic need. For example, the condition of a person's cardiovascular and pulmonary system is one of the major influencing factors for the person's adaptation in oxygenation need, while the condition of the gastrointestinal system is a major influencing factor for that person's nutritional need.

2. The significance of each influencing factor in relation to the behaviors assessed in the 1st level assessment – the cause and effect relationship which exists between the 1st and 2nd level assessment.

3. The negative stimuli which has already caused ineffective responses or will potentially cause future problems.

The ultimate purpose of 2nd level assessment is to identify the causative stimuli for the ineffective behaviors manifested in the 1st level assessment.

The Third Step
Defining the Client's Adaptation Problem:
Nursing Diagnosis

The Nursing Diagnosis is a statement that describes the person's actual or potential adaptation problem and it is derived from analysis of the 1st level and 2nd level assessments.

A nursing diagnosis according to the Roy Model nursing process is to include three (3) components:

1. The statement of the adaptation problem;

2. The manifesting behaviors indicating the problem; and

3. The causative stimuli.

In order to make an accurate nursing diagnosis, the student should go through the following two steps:

First, review all of the ineffective behaviors recognized in the 1st level assessment, and sort them out into clusters according to the presenting adaptation problems. For example, during the 1st level assessment of Mr. A's oxygenation need, many ineffective behaviors are recognized. From the many ineffective behaviors assessed, such a group of behaviors as 1) "Not being able to follow instructions," 2) "Congested breath sound," and 3) "Not being able to cough up pharyngeal secretions" form a cluster of behaviors indicating one nursing diagnosis. This particular cluster of behaviors indicate that Mr. A is not able to effectively clear his airways.

Ineffective airway clearance becomes an adaptation problem/ nursing diagnosis for Mr. A., since maintaining an adequate airway is an essential part of meeting the oxygenation need:

Second, by reviewing all of the negative stimuli recognized in the 2nd level assessment, identify the specific stimuli that directly or indirectly caused the particular cluster of ineffective behaviors/problems. If the 2nd level assessment of Mr. A's oxygenation need included "Bacterial Pneumonia," "Dehydration," "Frequent use of Morphine Injections," and "Age 82 years," one can readily see the cause and effect relationship that exists between the above cluster of behaviors (1st level assessment) and the stimuli (2nd level assessment):

"Bacterial Pneumonia" is considered the Focal Stimulus since it directly caused the behaviors, while "Dehydration" and "Frequent Use of Morphine" made the situation worse by contributing as the Contextual Stimuli. Residual Stimuli are the influencing factors, such as the person's age, culture or environment, etc., which may have affected the behaviors, but which cannot be readily validated.

In summing up, the nursing diagnosis for Mr. A's oxygenation need in this situation should read:

Dx: Inability to Maintain an Adequate Airway:

Manifested by:
a) Not being able to follow instructions
b) Not being able to cough up pharyngeal secretions
c) Congested chest sound

Due to:
1. Bacterial Pneumonia (Focal Stimulus)
2. Dehydration (Contextual Stimulus)
3. Frequent Use of Morphine (Contextual Stimulus)

The listing of the manifesting ineffective behaviors specific to the diagnosis is important in that it validates accuracy of the diagnosis.

Identifying the stimuli that are specific to the particular diagnosis is also important, because in the Roy Adaptation Model, the nursing intervention is done primarily by managing (manipulating) the specific stimuli that produce the ineffective behavioral responses. Therefore, careful examination of those specific stimuli and classification as *Focal, Contextual,* or *Residual* will be helpful in setting realistic nursing goals and formulating a proper nursing intervention.

A potential nursing diagnosis is made when the 1st level assessment does not identify any ineffective behaviors at the present time; however, the 2nd level assessment reveals strong negative stimuli which may cause a predictable adaptation problem. Identifying potential nursing diagnoses is important in that the problems can be prevented with proper nursing intervention in advance.

In making a nursing diagnosis, the student learns that:

1. A nursing diagnosis has to be supported by a correct set of manifesting ineffective behaviors and causative stimuli to demonstrate the logical cause and effect relationship.

2. A nursing diagnosis is not a medical condition (such as anemia, hypertension, or infection) but most likely it is the client's problem in dealing with the medical problems and other stimuli.

3. There are common adaptation problems in each basic need area and the nurse should work towards prevention of the problems. Common nursing diagnoses are listed in the assessment tool.

4. A potential diagnosis can be made even without obvious manifesting behaviors as long as there are specific negative stimuli which may cause a predictable adaptation problem.

The Fourth Step
Setting the Client's Nursing Goal

Goal setting is done by defining the anticipated behavioral outcome expected of the client in solving the adaptation problem(s) described by the particular nursing diagnosis. Each nursing diagnosis is to have its own nursing goal, and each goal is to have its own set of nursing interventions through which the goal would be accomplished.

A nursing goal should not be confused with a medical goal. A goal such as "The client will increase his Hgb. level to 14 mg." is not a nursing goal, since it requires, primarily, medical interventions to achieve it. A nursing goal should be achievable through nursing interventions that can be carried out by the nurse, independent of the medical interventions. A nursing goal should also be stated in such a way to directly reflect the nursing diagnosis. For example, if the nursing diagnosis were *"Ineffective Airway Clearance,"* the client's nursing goal would be, *"The client will maintain an Adequate Airway."*

At times, a nursing diagnosis may call for more than one nursing goal – a long term goal and a short term goal – depending on the nature and imminence of the problems presented. Let's examine the following situation:

Dx: Inadequate Bowel Elimination:

Manifested by:
   a) Absence of bowel movement for several days
   b) Evidence of lower bowel impaction
   c) Abdominal discomfort
   d) Poor appetite

In this situation, the diagnosis (with manifesting behaviors) calls for two nursing goals: an immediate goal and a long term goal. The immediate goal would be *"Will be relieved from the impacted bowel condition as soon as possible"* and it will require a nursing intervention which calls for prompt nursing action. The long term goal would be *"Will establish a regular bowel habit within a week"* and it will require nursing interventions which may include some planning for the teaching-learning process for behavior modification.

In setting a client's nursing goal, the student learns that:

1. A nursing goal is the expected outcome produced through implementation of the proposed nursing interventions.

2. The expected outcome should be stated in behavioral terms with a reasonable time frame, so that it can be measured.

3. A nursing goal should directly reflect the nursing diagnosis and be realistic in terms of the outcome and time frame.

The Fifth Step
Formulation of Nursing Interventions

Nursing interventions are those actions which will assist the client in accomplishing the set nursing goal by breaking the cause and effect chain reflected in the specific nursing diagnosis. In adaptation nursing, nursing interventions, most of the time, involve dealing directly with the specific stimuli listed under the nursing diagnosis. **While the positive stimuli are reinforced, the negative stimuli are removed, reduced, or changed. The purpose of managing the stimuli is to bring about changes in the cause (stimuli) and effect (ineffective behaviors) relationship described in the nursing diagnosis.**

Many times, especially when the Focal stimulus happens to be a medical condition, the list of nursing interventions may include carrying out some of the medical therapies already prescribed by the physician. For example, when the Focal stimulus for a nursing diagnosis happens to be Bacterial Pneumonia, the nursing intervention will include carrying out all the therapies prescribed by the physician for that condition, as well as dealing with other Contextual and Residual stimuli, which require independent nursing actions.

Successful outcome of nursing intervention depends upon the accuracy of the diagnosis, the person's general coping capability, and the number and seriousness of the negative stimuli the person is faced with at a given time.

In formulating and implementing nursing interventions, the student learns that:

1. The purpose of any proposed nursing intervention is to bring about changes by breaking the chain of cause (stimuli) and effect (response) indicated in the diagnosis.

2. Breaking the cause and effect chain is accomplished by dealing directly with each of the causative stimuli under the nursing diagnosis: removing, reducing, or changing the negative stimuli.

3. Each intervention should be directly or indirectly capable of producing the expected behavioral outcome prescribed in the goal statement.

The Sixth Step
Evaluation and Modification of the Nursing Intervention

Evaluation/modification is the last step of the nursing process. When implementation is completed, effectiveness of the nursing intervention should be evaluated: *Has the client's nursing goal been achieved? Did the interventions produce the expected outcome prescribed in the goal?*

Evaluation is done according to the expected behavioral outcome with the time frame prescribed in the goal statement: Demonstration of the expected behavior(s) by the client indicates successful outcome, while lack of demonstration indicates a less than successful outcome.

Unsuccessful outcome of nursing interventions can stem from three major reasons: 1) Inaccurate 1st and 2nd level assessment which led to an inaccurate diagnosis, and therefore dealing with the wrong stimuli; 2) Having an unrealistic goal that cannot be achieved by the nurse and client, and 3) Having too many and overwhelmingly serious stimuli to face at a given time. **When it is evident that the goal is obviously not achieved, the situation requires total re-assessment. Either start with a new diagnosis and stimuli or modify the intervention strategies, depending upon the reasons for failure.**

In the evaluation phase of the nursing process, the student learns that:

1. The behavioral outcome with a time frame prescribed in the goal statement is to be used as criteria for evaluation of the outcome.

2. The evaluation result determines future nursing action: no further action, modification of the intervention strategies, or return to the 1st and 2nd level assessment.

Assessment Categories

A Person as an Adaptive System with 4 Modes of Adaptation

Modes of Adaptation	Needs to be met	Sub components
Physiological Mode Responses to stimuli from the environment to meet the survival needs.	Biological Integrity	Basic needs and regulatory functions: - Oxygenation - Fluid and Electrolytes - Nutrition - Elimination - Rest and Activity - Neurosensory - Protection
Self Concept Mode Need to know who one is so that one can be and exist with a sense of unity.	Psychic Integrity	Physical Self: - Body image - Body sensation Personal Self: - Self-Consistency - Self Ideal - Moral-Ethical/Spiritual Self
Role Function Mode Need to know who one is in relation to others so that one can act (play the role) appropriately.	Social Integrity	Roles - Primary - Secondary - Tertiary Role Behavior - Instrumental - Expressive
Interdependence Mode Need to have close relationships to meet: - Affectional adequacy - Developmental adequacy - Resource adequacy	Relationship Integrity	Structural: - Significant others - Supportive systems Interactive: - Receptive - Contributive

According to the Roy Adaptation Model of nursing, the human person is a Bio-Psycho-Social being and functions as an adaptive system with four (4) modes of adaptation; namely, the Physiological, Self concept, Role Function and Interdependence mode. As a system, all four modes are connected to function as a whole in order to maintain its integrity, and it does so by virtue of interdependence among the four modes of adaptation. Therefore, one should keep in mind that rarely one mode alone would be affected by any stimuli. A given stimulus may produce multiple and rather complex responses involving more than one mode of adaptation. An adaptation problem in one mode would undoubtedly have an effect on other modes. A nursing diagnosis in one mode may serve as stimulus to behaviors in other modes. The beginning level students may be confused with the inter-modal (cross-modal) nature of the client's adaptation challenges. One way of avoiding the confusion is to make sure the nursing diagnosis and goal are focused on the specific need or mode being assessed, however complex the adaptation problems may seem to be. For example, if grieving over a significant other is one of the stimuli for poor eating behaviors in the Nutritional Need assessment, the nursing diagnosis is **"Inadequate Nutritional Intake"** and the list of nursing interventions would include assisting the person with the grieving process to achieve the expected outcome of increasing the person's nutritional intake. In the Self Concept mode, **"Grieving Over Loss of a Significant Other"** is the nursing diagnosis itself, and the expected outcome for any nursing intervention would be that the person will go through the grieving process successfully.

The beginning level students are encouraged to practice the assessment of each need/mode thoroughly first to learn the content of the 1st and 2nd level assessment and the common adaptation problems in each need/mode, then to carry out total assessment of a person for all four modes. An advanced student will be able to carry out a quick review of each need/mode without spending much time and recognize behaviors which call for a thorough assessment of certain specific need/mode.

Assessment of Physiological Mode

This assessment tool is developed according to the Basic Needs of the Roy Adaptation Model, which is different from the body system's approach of the medical model. The physiological mode includes seven (7) Basic Needs areas: Oxygenation, Fluid and Electrolyte Regulation, Nutrition, Elimination, Rest/Activity, Neurosensory Regulation, and Protection needs. These are considered basic to physiological survival. The Endocrine function need is not included in the list because, by its nature, it is integrated into all the basic needs as underlying stimuli for medical conditions.

How to Use the Tool

The First Column (**1st Level Assessment**), starting from the left, includes the list of representative behaviors that are to be assessed to check out whether the person's particular basic need is adequately met or not met at the present time. The student is to carry out the 1st level assessment according to this list. The right side of this column includes norms for each of the behaviors. The student is instructed to compare each of the assessed behaviors to these norms in order to recognize the ineffective behaviors. The presence of ineffective behaviors indicate possible adaptation problems.

The Second Column (**2nd Level Assessment**) has the list of Major Influencing Factors (stimuli) for Adaptation in the particular basic need. The student is to carry out the 2nd level assessment systematically according to this list. While assessing the stimuli, the student is to identify which stimuli are impinging as the negative stimuli in the particular need area at the present time for the client. Accurate assessment and identification of the negative stimuli are very important since nursing interventions are done by actively managing those negative stimuli and reinforcing the positive stimuli.

The Third Column (**Possible Nursing Diagnoses**) has the list of possible/common adaptation problems in the particular basic need area. The nursing diagnoses are formulated by analyzing the 1st level and 2nd level assessment data.

First, review the list of the nursing diagnoses in this column and compare them with the identified ineffective behaviors in the 1st level assessment. By doing so, the student will begin to see the correlations between a certain cluster of ineffective behaviors and a nursing diagnosis from the list. A cluster of ineffective behaviors indicates one of the diagnoses in the list. Then the diagnosis is made on the basis of the validating ineffective behaviors presented in the 1st level assessment. The student can also use the NADA list as long as the assessed behaviors logically reflect the diagnosis. A nursing diagnosis always has to be validated by a correct set of behaviors in order to be accurate.

Second, review all the negative stimuli identified in the 2nd level assessment and compare them with the ineffective behaviors listed under the diagnosis. By doing so, the student will begin to see the cause and effect relationship between a certain group of stimuli and the ineffective behaviors listed under the diagnosis. Then, understanding the cause and effect relationship, investigate which stimuli are impacting as Focal, Contextual, and Residual stimuli for the particular nursing diagnosis.

A nursing diagnosis with three (3) components will be indicated as follows:

Dx: Inadequate Caloric Intake

Manifested by:
   a) Daily minimum need = 1900 Cal > Actual intake = 500-800 Cal
   b) Under weighed by 40 lb.
   c) Complaints of being tired all the time

Due to:
   1. Nausea from Chemotherapy – F
   2. Poor appetite/very picky eater – C
   3. Self concept; does not see self as "underweight" – C
   3. Has to prepare and eat meals alone – R

It is very important for the student to keep in mind that **each diagnosis being selected has to be validated with a correct set of behaviors from the 1st level assessment, as well as with a particular set of stimuli from the 2nd level assessment.** The statement of diagnosis should reflect the cause and effect relationship between the cluster of behaviors and the stimuli.

Introduction to Oxygenation Need Assessment

The primary adaptation challenge of oxygenation need is in maintaining adequate oxygen balance at all times. This is because a human being's chance for survival without adequate O_2 is limited to a maximum of 3-4 minutes; that makes the oxygenation need the most important human basic need. Adequate O_2 balance is maintained when the O_2 delivery equals the constantly changing body's O_2 demand for adequate tissue perfusion.

This ability to maintain adequate O_2 balance is very much dependent upon the following four factors (stimuli). All the stimuli listed under the oxygenation need fall into one of these categories.

1. Adequate quality of air one breathes in

2. Effective functions of one's Cardio-Vascular-Pulmonary system

3. Adequacy of the circulatory volume and its concentration, particularly of the electrolytes and hemoglobin

4. Body's O_2 demand in a given time

Any abnormalities, disruptions, or drastic changes in any of these factors will negatively impact one's ability to maintain adequate O_2 balance and may cause ineffective behaviors in the 1st level assessment.

The samples of likely clusters of ineffective behaviors are listed on the next page, along with the list of possible nursing diagnoses. The student is, for practice, to match each group (cluster) of behaviors with a nursing diagnosis.

Manifesting Behaviors	Possible Nursing Diagnoses
A. Sudden change in mentation as the earliest sign of oxygen deficit; combative/irrational behaviors	• Inability to maintain an adequate airway • Ineffective breathing
B. Increase in the respiratory and pulse rates; labored breathing; complaints of S.O.B., weakness and dizziness; possibly experiencing slight chest pain	• Hyperventilation • Hypoventilation • Confusion/disorientation and potential for physical injury
C. Congested breath sound, but not able to handle respiratory secretions with effective cough	• Negative O_2 balance • Activity intolerance secondary to negative O_2 balance
D. Very shallow breathing with very little chest expansion	• Impending shock
E. Respiration < 9/min.	
F. Respiration > 30/min.	
G. Complaints of dizziness and fatigue during and following normal ADL, plus behaviors in B	
H. ↑ in pulse rate with ↓ in pulse strength and blood pressure accompanied by pale, cool, and clammy skin	

Oxygenation Need

1st Level Assessment	2nd Level Assessment	Possible Nursing Diagnoses
Assessment of Behaviors and Recognition of Ineffective Behaviors. Assess all according to the BASIC NEED area, then compare them to the norms in order to identify the Ineffective Behaviors.	Assessment of Influencing Factors and Identification of the Negative stimuli. Review all of the Common Influencing factors listed below in order to identify the specific Negative stimuli.	Identification of Adaptation Problems which can be validated by the Ineffective Behaviors in the 1st level assessment and caused by the specific stimuli identified in the 2nd level assessment.
Are there any ineffective behaviors?	Which of the following caused the ineffective behaviors?	Which of the following is validated by the 1st and 2nd level assessment?

BEHAVIORS	NORMS		
1. Early signs of O_2 deficit, change in:	1. No early signs of O_2 deficit:	I. Quality of the actual air one breathes in normally, via a mask or tube	**Potential or Actual Nursing Diagnoses:**
A. Level of consciousness	A. Able to respond appropriately to verbal commands as well as tactile stimuli. Gag reflex present. Able to cough up normal pharyngeal secretions.	II. **Presence of any pathophysiological conditions in the structures and functions responsible for the oxygenation process:** *Respiratory:* disease, obstruction or injury in the airway; lung and neuromuscular function such as COPD, Ca of the lung, pneumonia, paralysis, etc.	- Inability to maintain an adequate airway for physical injury - Confusion/disorientation with potential - Negative O_2 balance - Ineffective breathing - Hypoventilation - Hyperventilation - Activity intolerance secondary to negative O_2 balance - Self care knowledge deficit regarding O_2 need

		Cardiovascular: disease, obstruction or injury in the circulatory pumping and transportation systems such as arrhythmia, CHF, MI, arteriosclerosis, hypertension, embolism, stroke, etc.	Potential for collaborative nursing diagnosis:*
B. Behavior Pattern	B. No signs of confusion. Oriented to time, place, & person. Behaviors are rational		- Cardiovascular complications - Pulmonary complications - Impending shock - Hemorrhage
C. Sudden change in visual acuity as earliest sign of O_2 deficit	C. No signs that indicate sudden change in visual acuity	III. Changes in any of the following due to disruption in other body systems: - Vascular volume and content - Hemoglobin level - Fluid and Electrolyte balance	
D. Chest pain	D. No chest pain		
2. **Respiratory Pattern:**	2. **Respiratory Pattern:**	IV. Consumption of any of the following medications: - CNS depressant - Digitalis - Vasodilator or vasoconstrictor	
A. Rate	A. 16-24 norm for adult	V. Experiencing Pain at present time	
B. Type & Volume	B. Rhythmic, effortless	VI. Change in altitude and climate	
C. Chest movement	C. No apparent intercostal, sternal retractions or excessive use of scalenus/muscles	VII. Experiencing emotional excitement or stress and anxiety at present time	
D. Breath Sound	D. Clear without sounds of congestion	VIII. Poor nutritional condition that may affect O_2 status	*When there is no ineffective behaviors in the 1st level assessment, but there is a known medical condition which is being treated medically at present time.

(cont'd next page)

E. Subjective feelings of S.O.B.

F. Type and extent of pharyngeal secretion and ability to cough up

3. Circulatory Function:
A. Blood Pressure = $CO \times VR$

B. Pulse Rate and Regularity

C. Skin – color, warmth and moisture

D. Capillary Refill

4. Exercise Tolerance

5. Self care Knowledge about O_2 need

E. No complaints of "S.O.B." at rest

F. Able to cough up and handle secretions

3. Circulatory Function:
A. Systole 90-140 Diastole 60-90 with pulse pressure of 30-40

B. Rate: 60-90/M Regular and Full. No pulse deficits

C. Warm, Dry without clamminess, paleness or cyanosis

D. Returns within 3 second

4. Should not develop S.O.B., dizziness, fainting, or chest pain during or following usual daily living activities – pulse may increase 20-30 beats per min. with mild to moderate physical activity (50 hops on one foot) but it should return to normal within 2-3 mins.)

5. One should have adequate knowledge about diet, exercise, & other related factors

IX. Physical activity level: physical fitness

X. Conditions that require drastic increase in O_2 consumption such as:
- fever.
- sudden vigorous physical activity
- increase in basic metabolism

XI. Other health factors such as smoking, overweight which affect one's O_2 status

Notes:

Introduction to Fluid/Electrolyte Regulation Need Assessment

The primary adaptation challenge in meeting fluid/electrolyte need is in maintaining homeostasis in body fluid volume and its concentration of important electrolytes; net gain or net loss will cause imbalance. A human being's chance for survival without adequate fluid and electrolyte balance is limited to a few hours up to a maximum of a very few days. Therefore, the F/E regulation need is the second most important human basic need.

One's ability to maintain adequate F/E balance is dependent upon the following three major factors. All the stimuli listed under F/E regulation need assessment fall into one of these categories:

1. Effectiveness of one's GI system function for adequate ingestion, digestion, and absorption of fluid and electrolytes from the daily consumption of food and fluid.

2. Effectiveness of one's renal system for adequate filtration and secretion of excessive fluid, electrolyte and metabolic end products (effective cardiovascular function contributes to this cause).

3. Adequacy of fluid and electrolytes intake in replacement of fluid and electrolyte loss.

Any abnormalities, disruptions, or drastic changes in any of these factors will negatively impact one's ability to maintain adequate F/E balance and may cause ineffective behaviors in the 1st level assessment.

Samples of likely clusters of ineffective behaviors along with a list of possible nursing diagnoses are presented on the following page. The student is, for practice, to match each cluster of behaviors with an appropriate nursing diagnosis from the list.

Manifesting Behaviors	Possible Nursing Diagnoses

A. B.P. in sitting position is much less than lying B.P. with the difference greater than 15 mm Hg in systole and 10 mm Hg in diastole; ↓ urinary output	• Dehydration
	  - early stage
	  - advanced stage

B. Overnight ↑ in body weight of more than 1.5 lbs.	• Fluid overload
	  - early stage
	  - advanced stage

C. Behaviors in A, plus:
- ↓ B.P. below one's norm with ↑ pulse rate
- ↓ urinary output to a minimum (< 30 cc) with ↑ in concentration
- ↓ intraocular pressure
- Overnight ↑ in hemoconcentration without blood transfusion
- Very warm and dry skin with poor turgor
- Lack of neck vein filling in flat lying position without a pillow
- Other subjective and objective signs, such as fatigue, dizziness and listlessness, etc.
	• Electrolyte imbalance
	  - hypo
	  - hyper

D. Behavior in B, plus: - ↓ or absence of urinary output - Skin with presence of pitting edema - Exaggerated neck vein filling in lying position or evidence of neck vein filling with head elevation - ↑ B.P. to above the norm	
E. Abnormal electrolyte level	

Fluid & Electrolyte Need

1st Level Assessment	NORMS	2nd Level Assessment	Possible Nursing Diagnoses
BEHAVIORS			
1. Type and Amount of Urinary Output	**1. Type and Amount of Urinary Output:**	1. Presence of any pathophysiological conditions in the structure and functions responsible for maintaining body fluid and electrolyte balance:	Potential or Actual:
A. Color, concentration, and amount	A. Urine should be straw to slightly amber color and at a minimum rate of 30 cc/hr.	A. Conditions interfering with *Ingestion, Digestion, or Absorption of fluid and electrolytes:*	- **Dehydration:** *Early stage* *Advanced stage*
2. Body Weight Trend	**2. Body Weight Trend:**	- Disruption in the gastrointestinal system, including nausea	- **Fluid overload:*** *Early Stage* *Advanced Stage with susceptibility to tissue breakdown in the edematous area* *Difficulty in following instructions on fluid/diet restriction*
A. Gain – overnight gain as sign of fluid retention	A. Should be weighed at the same time each day with less than 0.5 lb. change (2 lb. gain = 1000 cc saline gain)	- Medically imposed N.P.O.	
3. Circulatory Status	**3. Circulatory Status:**	B. Conditions interfering with *excretion of excess body fluid, electrolyte and the metabolic end products. Such as:*	- **Electrolyte imbalance***
A. B.P. in different position (Orthostatic) – compare the sitting B.P. with the lying B.P. (for a sign of fluid volume deficit)	A. B.P. difference between B.P. in sitting position and lying position should be less than 15 mm Hg in Systole and 10 mm Hg in Diastole	- Renal disease	- **Self care knowledge deficit regarding maintenance of proper fluid and electrolyte balance**
B. Neck vein filling with elevated head position as sign of fluid volume overload (secondary to ineffective cardiac function)	B. No visible neck vein filling when head is elevated	- Cardiac insufficiency	*This diagnosis requires collaboration from the medical profession in planning the interventions
C. Pulse	C. Increase in pulse rate with drop in BP indicate fluid volume deficit	- Endocrine disturbances	**This diagnosis cannot be made without actual laboratory test results
		- Shock	

4. **Skin and Mucosa**
   A. Temperature
   B. Turgor
   C. Mucus Membrane
   D. Edema

5. **Intraocular Tension**

6. **Hemoconcentration** (sudden increase in Hgb. and HCT)

7. **Other signs of dehydration or fluid overload**

8. **Electrolyte Status:** A and B are not specific to Electrolyte status
   A. Change in Mentation and Affect
   B. Muscular tension
   C. Current serum electrolyte level

9. **Self care knowledge related to fluid and electrolyte balance**

---

4. **Skin and Mucosa:**
   A. Should not be hot or cold
   B. Good turgor
   C. Should be moist
   D. No pitting present

5. **Intraocular tension:** Should not look sunken or puffy

6. **Hemoconcentration:** Hgb. & Hct do not change overnight unless one has blood transfusion or hemorrhage

7. **Other general signs of dehydration,** such as dizziness, weakness, and headache, are not accompanied by other signs of fluid volume deficit

8. **Signs of electrolyte imbalance:**
   A. Should not show apathy or extreme nervousness
   B. There should be no muscular twitching or flaccidity
   C. Refer to textbook

9. **Should have sufficient knowledge & understanding of any dietary or fluid restrictions**

II. **Type and Amount of F/E intake:**
   - Enteral, Oral, and N/G or G tubes
   - Parenteral and other

III. **Type & Amount of F/E loss other than normal elimination:**
   - diarrhea, vomiting, or gastric suction
   - bleeding
   - secretion from wound/ burns or diaphoresis

IV. **Medication affecting F/E status:**
   - diuretics or antidiuretics
   - electrolytes

V. **Increase or decrease in the environmental temperature**

VI. **Other general conditions which may impede circulation:**
   - CHF
   - Tissue injuries
   - Obstructions

Introduction to Nutrition Need Assessment

There are two major adaptation challenges in nutrition need. The first is in maintaining adequate caloric balance for energy need and keeping adequate body weight. The second is in maintaining adequate intake of essential nutritional elements for healthy physiological processes such as growth, development, and repair of body tissues. A person's chance for survival without any nutritional intake is limited to days up to a maximum of not more than two weeks. Therefore, nutrition need is also one of the most important basic needs for survival.

One's ability to maintain adequate nutritional status is very much dependent upon the following factors. All the stimuli listed in the tool fall into one of these categories:

1. Effective functioning of the gastrointestinal system to ingest, digest, and absorb nutrients.

2. Availability and palatability of nutritional substances.

3. Metabolic, energy, growth, and repair needs in a given time.

4. Psychosocial factors involved in food and eating habits.

Any abnormalities, disruptions, or drastic changes in any of the above factors will negatively impact one's ability to meet one's nutritional need and may cause ineffective behaviors in the 1st level assessment.

Samples of likely clusters of ineffective behaviors along with a list of possible nursing diagnoses are presented on the following page. The student is, for practice, to match each cluster of behaviors with an appropriate nursing diagnosis from the list.

Manifesting Behaviors	Possible Nursing Diagnoses
A. Caloric intake < caloric need Decreasing trend in body weight Complaints of tiredness Other indirect signs such as: lack of hair density and luster, and poor skin integrity	• Inadequate caloric intake • Excessive caloric intake • Nutritional deficiency in *(specific elements)* • Altered means of nutritional intake
B. Caloric intake > caloric need Body weight above the ideal weight	
C. Food consumption lacking in variety to meet daily recommended intake of adequate *Carbohydrate, Protein, Fat, Fiber* and *minerals* with *vitamins*	
D. Use of Nasogastric or gastrostomy tubes for nutrition intake Use total parenteral nutrition	

Nutritional Need

1st Level Assessment	2nd Level Assessment	
BEHAVIORS	**NORMS**	**Possible Nursing Diagnoses**
		Potential or Actual:
1. Nutritional intake:	**1. Nutritional Intake:**	**I.** Presence of any pathophys-
A. Calorie intake vs. need	A. Total caloric intake should be	iological conditions in the
- Oral	equal to total caloric need	structures and functions
- Other means (TPN or tube		responsible for ingestion,
feedings - NG, G, J)	B. Consumes food from the 6	digestion, and absorption
B. Types of food consumed in	basic groups, meeting the	of fluid and food:
terms of 6 basic nutrients:	need for:	- Taste/smell sense
Bread group (6-11)	Protein	- Oral condition - mucosa, teeth
Meat group (2-3)	Carbohydrate	- Disruption in the GI system:
Fruit group (2-4)	Fat	surgery, Ca, inflammation,
Dairy group (2-3)	Mineral and vitamin	nausea obstruction, problems
Vegetable group (3-5)	Fiber	in digestive enzyme, etc.
Fat (sparingly)		**II. Other general disease and**
C. Dietary supplements	C. Takes adequate amount of	**illness conditions that**
	dietary supplements when	**require change in caloric**
	needed	**and dietary needs such as:**
2. Weight in Comparison to	**2. The person's current weight:**	- Hyper or hypothyroidism
Height:	Should be close to the ideal	- Diabetes mellitus
Ideal weight	weight – Allow 100 lbs. for	- Fever
Actual weight	5 ft. and add 5 lbs. to every	- Cardiovascular diseases
	inch above that; for males	- Obesity
	add 5-10 lbs. extra	

Additional diagnoses (right column):

- Inadequate caloric intake
- Nutritional deficiency in _____ (certain elements)
- Excessive caloric intake and potential for overweight
- Altered means (maintenance of) of nutritional intake: NG, G tubes or T.P.N.
- Difficulty in adjusting to dietary restrictions
- Self care knowledge deficit regarding nutrition

3. Integumentary Manifestation of Nutritional Status:

A. Skin texture and intactness

B. Density and texture of hair

C. Presence of wound that does not heal in time

4. **Subjective feelings of being "tired" and "weak":**

5. **Use of altered means of nutritional intake:**

A. Nasogastric tube feeding

B. TPN

C. Other IV infusions

6. **Self care knowledge about good nutritional intake:**

A. Basic knowledge

B. Dietary restrictions, if any

3. Integumentary Manifestation of Nutritional Status:

A. Skin should be smooth, not too thin, and free of unhealed wounds

B. Hair should be sufficient with volume showing luster

C. Wound healing within 1-2 weeks of injury

4. **Subjective feelings of being tired and weak** do not persist unless they are related to prolonged inactivity or oxygenation problem

5. **Altered means of nutritional intake** to meet nutrition need is not necessary, such as:
   - Tube feedings
   - TPN

6. **Self care knowledge:**

A. Person should have adequate knowledge about the 6 basic groups of food

B. Person understands own dietary restrictions and their importance in order to adhere to these restriction(s)

III Psychosocial Factors:
- Cultural practice
- Religious practice
- Economic conditions
- Self concept and Stress/Anxiety
- Eating environment
- Personal dietary habits

IV. Factors affecting appetite:
- Physical activity vs. Inactivity
- Palatability - likes & dislikes
- Poor environment
- Emotional or physical stress

V. **Change in Metabolic Rate which requires change in Caloric need:**
- Pregnancy
- Age – Growing vs. Aging stage
- Sedentary vs. Active lifestyle

VI. **Medications affecting one's nutritional status:**
- Corticosteroids therapy
- Insulin therapy
- Appetite controller
- Others

Introduction to Solid Elimination Need Assessment

Regular elimination of bowel waste is one of the normal body functions essential to one's health and sense of well-being. Any disruptions in the function will have systemic effect on one's health. Therefore, the adaptation challenge of solid elimination is in maintaining healthy bowel habits to meet the solid elimination need. One's ability to maintain adequate bowel elimination function is dependent upon the following major factors. All the stimuli listed under the solid elimination need fall into one of these categories:

1. Effective function of the gastrointestinal system, especially of the lower bowel.

2. Adequacy of the quantity and quality of residue in the diet.

3. Maintenance of adequate gastric motility.

4. Adequate daily fluid intake.

5. Absence of irritating chemicals or food substances, and inflammations in the intestinal tract which may interfere with normal bowel function.

6. Psycho-socio-cultural factors related to bowel habits.

Any abnormalities, disruptions, or drastic changes in any of the above factors will negatively impact one's ability to meet one's bowel elimination need and may cause ineffective behaviors in the 1st level assessment.

Samples of likely combinations of ineffective behaviors for an appropriate nursing diagnosis are listed on the following page, along with the list of possible nursing diagnoses.

Manifesting Behaviors	Possible Nursing Diagnoses

A. Small and dry stool which is difficult to expel
 	
Feelings of "not satisfied" or "not completed" with feeling of bloatedness
	• Discomfort of flatulence
	
	• Inadequate bowel elimination
	  - constipation
	  - fecal impaction

B. Continuous leakage of small amount of liquid (stool)
 	
Palpable mass in the left lower quadrant of abdomen
 	
Hard mass on digital rectal examination
 	
Sluggish bowel sounds
	• Problems associated with excessive bowel elimination:
	  - discomfort
	  - loss of body F/E and nutrients
	  - cross contamination, if there's any broken skins near by

C. Distended abdomen with feelings of bloatedness Intermittent but sharp abdominal pain ↑ resonance on percussion Absence or difficulty in expelling flatus	• Altered means of elimination
D. Abdominal cramps Consecutive frequent unformed/watery stools	
E. Has colostomy or ileostomy	

Solid Elimination Need

BEHAVIORS	NORMS	2nd Level Assessment	Possible Nursing Diagnoses
1st Level Assessment			
1. Characteristics of bowel elimination:	**1. Characteristics of bowel elimination:**	I. **Presence of any Patho-physiological conditions in the structures and functions responsible for formation and excretion of fecal waste:**	Potential or Actual:
A. Amount	A. & B. Should not be in a very small amount with increased frequency (not more than 2-3x a day - not less than 1x every 2-3 days)		- **Inadequate bowel elimina-tion:**
B. Frequency			*Constipation*
			Fecal impaction
C. Color	C. Brown; free from bloody stain or black, tarry appearance	- GI System – obstruction, inflammation, surgery, and others	
D. Consistency, shape, and easiness in expelling with sense of satisfaction or "Completeness"	D. Soft/formed or semi-formed, should not have difficulty in expelling	- Neurosensory disruption – paralysis, unconsciousness, and others	- **Problems associated with Excessive Bowel Elimination:***
			Discomfort
			Cross-contamination
2. Abdomen – Presence of:	**2. Abdomen** should be soft, flat without palpable mass. There should be bowel sounds every 10-15 sec-onds. One should be free from discomfort/pain or feeling of bloatedness	II. **Amount and type of food and fluid intake in the daily diet:**	*Loss of body F/E & nutrients*
A. distention		- bulk and fiber	
B. intermittent sharp pain		- fluid	- **Discomfort of flatulence**
C. feeling of "fullness"		III. **Adequacy in daily physical activity level**	
D. sluggish bowel sound			- **Altered means (maintenance of) of bowel elimination**
E. palpable fecal mass		IV. **Medications:**	
F. increased resonance on per-cussion		- CNS depressant	- **Self care knowledge deficit regarding solid elimination need**
		- Cathartics or Anticathartics	

3. Use of altered means of elimination
A. colostomy
B. ileostomy

4. **Other:**
- headache
- malaise
- anorexia
- furred tongue
- lethargy

5. Knowledge about proper diet and exercise related to solid elimination

---

3. **Altered means of elimination:** Should be managed properly to maintain the function and skin integrity

4. **Check for fecal impaction,** if some of these behaviors are accompanied with absence of bowel movements

5. **One should have sufficient knowledge about diet, fluid and physical activity levels that promote normal bowel elimination**

V. External Factors:
- Available and suitable toilet facilities and assistance if needed
- Adequacy of privacy

VI. Other:
- General physical, mental, emotional condition
- Cultural or social customs, attitudes, and habits

---

*Diarrhea itself is not a nursing diagnosis but a symptom for many different medical conditions. Therefore, it is considered as stimulus for problems in other basic needs. It is an example of cross or inter-modal situations.

Introduction to Fluid Elimination Need Assessment

Since urine is being constantly produced by the kidney(s), it has to be collected in the bladder until released voluntarily. This process of transport, storage and voluntary release of urine is one of the bodily functions essential to one's health. Any disruption in this process would be detrimental to one's health. Therefore, the adaptation challenge of urinary elimination is in maintaining the process. One's ability to maintain the normal process of urinary elimination is dependent upon the following major factors. The stimuli listed in the tool fall into one of these categories:

1. Effective function of the lower urinary tract with its neurosensory function.

2. Urinary production by the kidney(s).

3. Psychosocial aspect related to one's urinary elimination habits.

4. Growth and developmental stage.

Any abnormalities, disruptions, or drastic changes in these factors will negatively impact one's ability to meet urinary elimination need and may cause ineffective behaviors in the 1st level assessment.

The samples of likely combinations of ineffective behaviors for an appropriate nursing diagnosis are listed on the following page, along with the list of possible nursing diagnoses.

Manifesting Behaviors	Possible Nursing Diagnoses

A. Very frequent voiding of a small amount with continuing urgency
Abdominal discomfort
Palpable bladder distention
Prolonged micturition effort to void
	• Loss of urinary control
	  - urinary incontinence
	  - urinary retention
	
	• Dysuria secondary to urinary tract infection or irritation

B. Very frequent or continuous involuntary voiding No palpable bladder distention No abdominal discomfort	• Potential for urinary tract infection • Altered means of urinary elimination
C. Continuous urgency Lower abdominal discomfort Burning sensation upon urination ↑ in temperature (may or may not be present)	
D. Poor personal hygiene in the genitourinary area Use of urinary catheter	
E. Use of urinary diversion: catheter, urostomy, or Kock pouch	

Fluid Elimination Need

1st Level Assessment	NORMS	2nd Level Assessment	Possible Nursing Diagnoses
BEHAVIORS			
1. Characteristics of micturition:	1. Characteristics of normal micturition:	I. Presence of any Patho-physiological conditions in the structures and functions responsible for normal micturition:	Potential or Actual:

A. Frequency, amount per voiding and control	A. Varies; normal bladder is able to hold urine 3-8 hrs. Increased frequency with less than 100 cc per voiding is not normal	- Infection
		- Obstruction
		- Neurotransmission problems
		- Injury
			- Loss of Urinary Control: *Urinary Incontinence* and related problems; effects on:
			  Skin integrity
			  Self concept
			  Urinary Retention

B. Sensation related to urination - Continuous urgency - Pain (burning sensation) with voiding - Lower abdominal discomfort - Need for straining to void	B. Normal micturition process begins, with intention, spontaneously and completes approximately within one minute without local pain or lower abdominal discomfort but with complete relief	II. Any condition interfering with the normal voiding process such as: - Pelvic surgery - Neurosensory disturbances - Anesthesia - Removal of catheter after a prolonged use	- Dysuria - Urinary tract infection - Altered means (maintenance of) of urinary elimination
C. Color D. Odor, clarity	C. Straw to slightly amber D. Clear & slightly aromatic without offending odor (upon voiding)	III. Increased vs. decreased urinary production secondary to:** - Fluid intake	- Self care knowledge deficit regarding bladder elimination need
E. Presence or absence of bladder distention	E. No signs of bladder distention upon abdominal palpation		

2. General:
A. Vital signs, particularly of signs of inflammation.

B. Personal hygiene.

3. Altered means of elimination:
- use of indwelling catheter(s)
- urostomy
- Kock pouch

4. Self care knowledge about maintaining good bladder elimination

2. General:
A. Should not have a sudden increase in body temperature associated with burning sensation upon urination

B. Poor hygiene promotes infection

3. Person should understand the situation, and if it is a permanent one should learn the care and maintenance of the altered means

4. One should have sufficient knowledge about the health practices related bladder elimination need

- Renal function
- Fluid loss via other route

IV. Growth and developmental stage:
- Age
- Sex

V. Other general mental and psycho-socio-environmental factors:
- Availability of suitable toilet and privacy facility and privacy
- Emotional condition – stress/anxiety level
- Mental status

*Fluid elimination need is restricted to the function of the lower urinary tract. It does not include fluid and electrolyte need.

Introduction to Rest and Activity Need Assessment

Physical activity not only allows one to carry out the daily survival chores, but also activates one's internal physiological processes; normal growth and development, maintenance of muscle tone/bone matrix, and hormonal activities are all dependent upon adequate physical stimulation. On the other hand, rest allows one's physiological process the time to restore and repair body tissues and functions.

Though the needed amounts of rest and activity vary from person to person, time to time, and situation to situation, one's rest and activity needs are dependent upon the following major factors. Most of the stimuli listed in the Rest and Activity need assessment fall into one of these categories:

1. Effective function of the neuro-musculo-skeletal systems.

2. General physical conditions such as nutrition, stress, disease and illness.

3. Psychological conditions and extent of psychological stress.

4. Socio-environmental factors related to activity and sleep habits.

5. Growth and developmental stage.

Any abnormalities, disruptions, or drastic changes in any of these factors will negatively impact one's rest and activity need and may cause ineffective behaviors in the 1st level assessment.

The samples of likely clusters of ineffective behaviors along with a list of possible nursing diagnoses are presented on the following page. The student is, for practice, to match each cluster with an appropriate nursing diagnosis.

Manifesting Behaviors	Possible Nursing Diagnoses
A. Subjective feeling of not being able to fall asleep and stay asleep	• Disuse syndrome
	• Inadequate physical activity/ potential for development of disuse effect

B. Very short night sleep period
Complaints of:
    tiredness, restlessness, sleepiness
    lack of concentration	

	• Activity intolerance/potential for physical injury
	• Total sleep deprivation
C. Frequent disruptions of sleep cycles, plus behaviors listed in B	• REM sleep deprivation
	• Insomnia
D. On complete bedrest or very little physical activity	
E. Loss of muscle mass, limited ROM and other disuse phenomena	
F. Lack of strength, coordination and speed – inability to sustain steady gait and erect posture	

Rest and Activity Need – Rest Need

BEHAVIORS 1st Level Assessment	NORMS 2nd Level Assessment	Possible Nursing Diagnoses
1. Quantity & Quality of Rest	**1. Quantity & quality of rest needed** are dependent upon individual's physical and emotional condition:	Potential or Actual:

A. Complaints of being unable to fall asleep	A. Has usual bedtime rituals and able to fall asleep without difficulties	- Insomnia
		
		- **Sleep deprivation:**
		   Total sleep deprivation
		   REM sleep deprivation

B. Complaints of being unable to stay asleep for the night	B. Once the person falls asleep, usually stays asleep for most of night without frequent/ long awake periods	
C. Sleep pattern: - Duration of sleep - number of arousals during sleep - Usual bedtime vs. Current bedtime - Quality of sleep	C. Average adult needs 6-8 hrs. of sleep per day with less than 1-2 interruptions, in order to feel rested. Change in bedtime may disturb the quality of sleep	
D. Nap or rest period - Number of - Quality of	D. Elderly or ill person needs 1 or 2 naps (or complete rest periods) due to deteriorated sleep quality	
	I. **Cortical activity level:** - stress - anxiety - fear	
	II. **General physical condition:** - Illness and disease - Trauma and stress - Pain experience - Nutrition status	
	III. **External environment:** - familiarity of environment - climate - amount & type of stimuli	
	IV. **Daily activity routine:** - Physical activity level - Personal habit or rest & activity cycle - Bedtime ritual	

BEHAVIORS	NORMS	2nd Level Assessment	Possible Nursing Diagnoses
2. Subjective feelings of: - "Tired" - "Restless" - "Sleepy" - "Nervous" 3. Signs of sleep deprivation: - Irritability - Frequent yawning - Inability to concentrate - Other	2. Subjective feelings should include "well rested" and "full of energy" regardless of the number of hours spent for sleep and rest 3. Well rested person will not demonstrate these objective signs	V. Developmental stage/age VI. Use of drugs and alcohol: - Stimulants - Sedatives	

Rest and Activity Need – Activity Need

BEHAVIORS	1st Level Assessment NORMS	2nd Level Assessment	Possible Nursing Diagnoses
1. Type and extent of medically imposed therapeutic restriction: - Complete bed rest - Bathroom privilege 2. Quality/quantity of physical exercise performed daily	1. Therapeutic restrictions are usually temporary, and as the medical condition improves, the restrictions should be reevaluated 2. Quality/quantity of daily physical activity are dependent upon the person's lifestyle; however, minimum of 20-30 min. daily exercise, beside the usual ADL, is recommended	I. Disease, trauma or deformity in neuro-musculo-skeletal system II. Other medical conditions requiring therapeutic restriction III. Lifestyle: Psychosocial aspect: - age - personality - habits - time availability	Potential or Actual: - Disuse syndrome - Inadequate physical activity/potential for disuse effect - Activity intolerance/potential for physical injury secondary to decreased physical stamina

(cont'd next page)

3. Signs/symptoms of disuse:

A. Type and extent of impairment in motor function, if any

B. Neuro-musculo-skeletal structure and function:
- Muscle mass for tone and strength
- Ranges of joint motions
- Posture and gait
- Coordination and balance

C. Other systemic effects of decreased physical activity

D. Physical stamina

4. Knowledge about activity need

3. No signs/symptoms of disuse:

A. Body movement should demonstrate usual speed and accuracy

B. Neuro-musculo-skeletal function
- Firm muscle mass with adequate volume and contractibility
- Full range of motion in all joints without pain
- Coordinated body movement with steady gait, erect body posture and adequate speed

C. Refer to textbook

D. Should be able to endure usual ADL activity and more without exhaustion

4. **One should know the benefits of regular exercise and physical fitness**

- access to suitable environment for physical exercise
- self concept/motivation
- value placed on physical fitness

IV. **Availability of personal assistance or assistive devices when needed**

V. **Prolonged physical inactivity**

VI. **Psychiatric disorders:**
- major depression
- catatonic state

Notes:

Introduction to Neurosensory Regulation Need Assessment

Sensory regulation need involves one's ability to receive, perceive, and react appropriately to ever-changing stimuli that one encounters in every moment of life. The ability to receive, perceive, and react is developed and maintained through continuous exposure to a variety of stimuli appropriate to the person's developmental stage. Inability to receive stimuli by the sensory receptors, perceive the stimuli correctly by the brain, or react appropriately by the musculoskeletal and other muscles will have a most detrimental impact on one's life. Therefore, neurosensory regulation is considered a basic function for survival.

One's ability to maintain adequate neurosensory function is dependent upon the following factors. All the stimuli listed under the neurosensory regulation need fall into one of these categories:

1. Effective function of the neurosensory organs: the sensory receptors, spinothalamic tract, and the brain.

2. Adequacy of sensory stimulation.

3. General physical and psychological condition.

4. Growth and developmental stage.

Any abnormalities, disruptions, or drastic changes in any of these factors will negatively impact one's ability to meet the sensory regulation need and may cause ineffective behaviors in the 1st level assessment.

The samples of likely clusters of ineffective behaviors along with a list of possible nursing diagnoses are presented on the next page. The student is, for practice, to match each of the clusters with an appropriate nursing diagnosis.

Manifesting Behaviors	Possible Nursing Diagnoses

A. Inappropriate responses to various stimuli
A Glasgow Coma Scale score of less than 15
	• Problems associated with neurosensory deficit:
	  - Confusion/disorientation
	  - Potential for physical injury
	  - Difficulty in carrying out ADL
	  - Difficulty in communication
	  - Learning to live with a sensory deficit

B. Behaviors in A, plus deficit in motor status	
C. Presence of receptive or expressive aphasia	
D. Deficit in one or more sensory receptors Change in affect ↓ in intellectual capacity	• Sensory perceptual deprivation • Sensory perceptual overload*
*E. Sudden confusion and disorientation Inability to make simple decisions Difficulty in abstract thinking No obvious known sensory deficit	• Pain • Discomfort of aberrant sensation
F. Complaints of pain sensation	
G. Complaints of abnormal sensations	
H. Permanent deficit in one or more sensory receptors	

* Associated with the quantity and quality of stimuli

Neurosensory Regulation Need

BEHAVIORS	NORMS	2nd Level Assessment	Possible Nursing Diagnoses
1st Level Assessment			
			Potential or Actual:
1. Mental Status:	**1. Mental Status:**	I. Presence of any patho-	- **Problems associated with**
A. Levels of Consciousness:	A. Awake, alert and respond-	physiological conditions	**neurosensory deficit:**
- Alert, wakeful	ing to all types of stimuli,	in the structures and func-	*Confusion/disorientation*
- Drowsy	including verbal command,	tions responsible for neu-	*Potential for physical injury*
- Stuporous	appropriately	rosensory regulation:	*Inability to carry out ADL*
- Comatose		- Sensory receptors –	*Difficulty in communication*
		peripheral nerves and 5	*Adjusting to living with senso-*
B. Glasgow Coma Scale:	B. Glasgow Coma Scale:	sensory modes	*ry limitations*
a. Eyes opening: 1-4 points	a. open eyes spontaneously	- Transmission path –	
b. Verbal response: 1-5 points	b. oriented to time, person and	spinothalamic tract	- Sensory perceptual overload
c. Motor response: 1-6 points	place	- Perceptor – brain	
	c. obeys orders appropriately	- Other conditions affecting	
7 or less is classified as comatose	*Total Score of 15 points*		
		II. Adequacy of sensory stim-	- Sensory perceptual depriva-
C. Behavior and appearance	C. Appearance and response	uli:	tion
(moods, hygiene, groom-	to environmental stimuli	- Intensity	
ing, body language)	should be appropriate	- Pattern	- Pain
		- Variety	
D. Presence of Aphasia:	D. Should be able to under-	- Appropriateness to the per-	- Discomfort of pruritus
Receptive Expressive	stand and express in famil-	son's growth/development	
	iar language		
E. Intellectual Function:	E. Demonstrate appropriate	III. Growth and development	
- memory	level to past experience,	level of the person	
- knowledge	educational and cultural		

- abstract thinking
- judgement

2. **Sensory Status**
A. *Visual*
- acuity   - known deficits
- corrective devices
- unusual sensations
B. *Auditory*
- ability to distinguish voices
- known deficits
- corrective devices
- unusual sensations
C. *Olfactory*
- ability to discriminate odors
- unusual sensations
D. *Gustatory*
- ability to discriminate sweet, sour, salty, bitter
- unusual sensations
E. *Tactile*
- ability to discriminate sharp, dull, light, firm touches
- unusual sensations
F. *Aberrant Sensation:* Pain, numbness, itching

3. **Motor Status**
- ability to move   - balance
- coordination   - reflexes

---

2. **Sensory Status**
A. Able to distinguish shape, color & distance of object one is looking at; let patient use corrective devices, such as glasses.
B. Able to distinguish different sounds, including voices.
C. Able to discriminate odors. (Use meal time for this assessment).
D. Able to discriminate different taste of different foods.
E. Able to distinguish different temperatures, sharpness or firmness of objects. Should be able to identify the part of body touched by an object.
F. Free from abnormal sensation: pain, numbness, or pruritus.

3. **Motor status** demonstrates well coordinated movement of body and extremities with adequate speed and strength without any difficulties.

IV. **General physical, mental and emotional condition**

V. **Physical injuries to musculoskeletal system/sensory organs**

VI. **Medications which may interfere with reception, perception, or reaction process**

Introduction to Protection Need Assessment

The three major modalities of protection include the immune, integumentary and neurosensory/motor functions. The integumentary system serves as the first line defense against externally-generated harmful stimuli such as chemicals, heat, physical trauma and microorganisms. An intact neurosensory system protects the person by enabling the person to receive, perceive, and react appropriately to the internal as well as external stimuli one is challenged with. The motor function enables the person carry out the reactions the brain commands. Finally, the immune system protects one's internal environment by neutralizing, eliminating, or destroying the invading microorganism and foreign elements. The adaptation challenge of the protection need is in maintaining adequate protective functions.

One's ability to meet protection need is dependent upon the following major factors. All the stimuli listed under the protection need fall into one of these categories:

1. Effective functioning of the Immune, Integumentary, Neurosensory, and Motor Function systems.

2. Good general physical and psychological condition and manageable stress level.

3. A healthy living internal and external environment.

Any abnormalities, disruptions, or drastic changes in any of these factors will negatively impact one's ability to meet protection need and may cause ineffective behaviors in the 1st level assessment.

The samples of clusters of ineffective behaviors along with a list of possible nursing diagnoses are presented on the next page. The student is, for practice, to match each cluster with an appropriate nursing diagnosis from the list.

Manifesting Behaviors	Possible Nursing Diagnoses
A. Frequent, multiple sites, or recurrent episodes of infection Inability to maintain adequate WBC level Poor response to antibiotic treatment B. Unhealthy integumentary system: - Compromised integrity in the integumentary system - Poor hygiene, poor circulation C. Deficit in motor function: - Inadequate speed - Lack of accuracy - Lack of strength D. Inability to receive, perceive or react to stimuli	• Inability to maintain physical safety • The effects of Impaired immune responses • Impaired skin integrity/potential for secondary infection or pressure sores

Protection Need

BEHAVIORS	NORMS		Possible Nursing Diagnoses
1st Level Assessment	NORMS	2nd Level Assessment	Possible Nursing Diagnoses
1. Specific to immune function:	**1. Specific to immune function:**	I. Presence of any pathophysiological conditions in the structures and functions responsible for immune response, such as:	Potential or Actual
A. Signs of immunodeficiency; Frequent or recurrent infection:	A. Person with good immune function will not be subject to frequent infections in usual environmental exposure. And the recovery would be uneventful.	- Bone marrow - Lymphoid tissues - Spleen - Other hematological factors	- Effect of impaired immune response
- Respiratory - Gastrointestinal - Skin and mucosa			
- Systemic manifestation with fever and chills		II. AIDS/HIV infection	
B. Lab findings: - Ability to maintain effective WBC count	B. Lab findings: WBC 5,000-10,000/mm^3 with differential neutrophils 1,500-7,500/mm^3	III. Immunosuppressive therapies for transplanted organ(s)	
- Poor response to antibiotic therapy		IV. Chemo/radiation therapy for neoplastic diseases	
2. Specific to physical safety: *Neurosensory* – Ability to	**2. Specific to physical safety:** *Neurosensory* Demonstrates appropriate responses to all types of stimuli that are internally generated as well as the externally generated stimuli.	V. Environmental exposures	
- Receive - Perceive		VI. Nutritional status	
- React to all types of stimuli		VII. Stress level	

09

Motor function
- Speed
- Accuracy/Coordination
- Strength

3. Specific to integumentary protection:

A. Skin texture and strength
- thickness
- elasticity
- dryness/wetness
- condition of areas with bony prominences
- hair growth

B. Hygiene
- cleanliness
- odor

C. Sensory response
- response to external stimuli: touch, heat, cold, pain and pleasure
- pruritus

D. Intactness
Presence of any possible and actual open lesions
- location
- type/depth

(cont'd next page)

Motor function
Able to complete body movements with accuracy, adequate strength and speed without any difficulties.

3. Specific to integumentary protection:

A. Skin surface should be smooth without transparent looks, but with signs of hair. It should be dry but not scaly with cracking appearance. There should be no skin areas continuously exposed to wetness.

B. Regular and good hygiene makes the skin free from contamination and odor.

C. Skin serves as a sensory receptor which will produce an appropriate reaction to harmful stimuli.

D. Skin as the container of internal organs and first line of defense should not have open lesions or

I. Presence of any pathophysiological conditions in the structure and functions responsible for effective body movements:
- Disruption in the neurosensory regulation system
- Disruption in the motor function

I. Disruption in the integumentary system function:
- Injuries/traumas
- Allergic reactions
- Manifestations of disease
- Inflammation/infection

II. General nutrition/hydration status

III. Mental status (self-care capability)

IV. Effects of immobility

V. Neuropathy

VI. Effects of Circulatory impairment

- Inability to maintain physical safety

- Impaired skin integrity and secondary infection

- Development of pressure sores and secondary infection

- size
- signs of infections
E. Self-care knowledge relative to skin care

injuries which may interfere with normal function.
E. One should be knowledgeable about the importance of skin as a protective organ and proper skin care.

- Fecal
- Urinary
- Irritants

General skin assessment related to other physiological functions

			Refer to the appropriate Basic Need.
4. Integumentary manifestation of other diseases and illness:	4. Integumentary manifestation of other disease and illness:	I. Disruption in various body functions and organs:	

4. Integumentary manifestation of other diseases and illness:

A. Color, warmth and moisture
B. Turgor
C. Presence of abnormal lesions or rashes.
- location/distribution
- characteristics
D. Aberrant sensations
E. Signs of local inflammation

4. Integumentary manifestation of other disease and illness:

A, B, C, D, & E: Health Person's skin is usually dry, warm and with good turgor

It should be free of:
- pallor
- cyanosis
- jaundice
- ecchymosis or purpura
- abnormal lesions or rashes
- aberrant sensations such as:
    pruritus
    pain
    heat
    numbness

I. Disruption in various body functions and organs:
- cardiovascular/pulmonary diseases
- anemia
- liver and other
- renal dysfunction
- local/systemic fungal, bacterial and viral infections
- allergies

Refer to the appropriate Basic Need.

Introduction to Assessment of Psychosocial Modes of Adaptation

Psychosocial Modes of Adaptation

According to the Roy Adaptation Model of nursing, one's psychosocial needs are met through three adaptation modes. They are the Self Concept, Role Function and Interdependence modes:

The Self Concept mode focuses on the person's psychological and spiritual aspects. The underlying basic need is the **psychic integrity** – the need to know "who one is so that one exist with a sense of unity."

The Role Function mode focuses on the roles one occupies in the society and how well the person carries out the set of expectations given to those roles. The underlying basic need is the **social integrity** – the need to know "who one is in relation to others so that one can act."

The Interdependence mode focuses on the close relationships of the person through which one's affectional adequacy, developmental adequacy and resource adequacy needs are met. The underlying basic need is the **relational integrity**.

Criteria for Judgment for Psychosocial Adaptation

Just as in the physiological mode, assessment of behaviors in the psychosocial modes need criteria for judgment. The criteria has to be the societal norms which are acceptable to most people in the society. The psychosocial developmental norms identified for each stage of life are used as the criteria because they are considered to be the socio-cultural norms of a society.

The developmental tasks one is to accomplish in a given stage of life mostly dictates the behaviors related to the person's psychosocial adaptation. How one feels about oneself, what kind of roles one occupies, how one plays out those roles, and what kind of relationships one develops and maintains are directly related to the stage of life the person is in. Therefore, the person's developmental stage is considered to be the most important influencing factor (stimulus) for the person's psychosocial adaptation in a given time. For an example, it is obvious that the role expectations of a 5-year-old child, in relation to the role of the child's parent, are quite different when the person becomes a 45-year-old child to the parent.

The following section of the tool presents the major developmental tasks for each stage of life and their relationships to the role functions, self concept and interdependence modes.

Using those criteria, the student is to keep in mind that these norms are very general to allow individual variations, yet they can be very specific according to a given culture.

The developmental norms are compiled from the following sources:

1. Erikson's stages of adult development.

2. Havighurst's developmental tasks.

3. Stevenson's developmental tasks for the four stages of adulthood.

Assessment Steps for Psychosocial Mode of Adaptation

Step 1 - Identify the person's age and developmental stage

Step 2 - Review the developmental tasks the client is to accomplish in that particular stage of life and set the criteria for judgment by finding out:

Role Function mode – what kinds of roles the person is suppose to occupy
Self Concept mode – how one usually feels about oneself
Interdependence mode – what kind of relationships one develops

Step 3 - Proceed with the nursing process using the specific tool provided

Developmental Norms as Criteria for Assessment of Psychosocial Mode of Adaptation

Stage of Life and Developmental Task	Usual Roles to Occupy	Self Concept	Interdependence
INFANCY **Trust vs. Mistrust** Through the loving and affectionate nurturing given, the child begins to develop a sense of trust.	- Child - Grandchild - Younger sister or brother	**Self concept is not formed yet.** Child does not feel self is separate from the caregiver and environment.	**Bonding → Attachment** with primary nurturer. Through this process, the sense of trust develops.
TODDLER YEARS **Autonomy vs. Shame/Doubt** As neuromuscular coordination development progresses, the child is able to exercise will power.	- Child - Grandchild - Younger or older sister or brother	**Begins to form self concept.** Through Separation and Individuation process, the child sees self as a separate being and "I," "me," "mine" and "no" are the first set of vocabulary used.	Goes through **Separation & Individuation.** By 2-3 years, child has **Intrapsychic Image** of significant others. This enables child to sense existence of others without their physical presence.
PRESCHOOL **Initiative vs. Guilt** Through socialization of playing with other children, the child learns not only to plan, initiate and undertake activities but also to follow rules and regulations in an environment other than own home.	- Same as above - Nursery school student - Friend	**Gender identification** becomes clear and child begins to emulate gender role behaviors. Beginning development of **Moral, Ethical, and Spiritual Self.**	The nature of friendship progresses: **Monetary Playmate → One-way Assistance.**

(cont'd next page)

SCHOOL YEARS **Industriousness vs. Inferiority** A sense of being competent is gained by working hard at school work and earning the passing grade. Work before play becomes an important factor in life as working hard and accomplishing given tasks are met with tangible outcomes.	- Student - Part time entrepreneur - Friend	**Self Ideal** begins to develop. Feels physically and mentally competent to carry out usual youth activities.	The nature of friendship progresses: **One-way Assistance** → **Two-way Fairweather Cooperation.**
ADOLESCENT YEARS **Self Identity vs. Identity Crisis and Role Confusion** Due to rapid physical change, growing peer competition, and social expectation, child goes through tremendous adaptation. Setting future career goals is dependent upon establishing an adequate self identity.	- Student - Part time employee - Special friend - Significant other	**Self definition** is developed through various activities and memberships in special activity groups. **Own sexuality** is being developed as beginning to be aware of own sexual orientation.	The nature of friendship takes the form of **Intimacy, Mutuality, and Sharing.** By the age of 15 yrs. and thereafter, one can develop and maintain **Autonomous and Interdependent** relationships.
YOUNG ADULTS IN TRANSITIONAL PERIOD: **(18-25 yrs.)** The primary objective is to establish one's self as an independent individual.			

1. Selects and prepares for a vocation.	- Student - Apprentice - Employee - Homemaker	**One has formed an Adequate Self Concept though it may be modified.** Following a successful completion of the adolescent years, one is able to answer "Who am I?" However, it is modifiable. *Physical Self* – Sees self as capable of carrying out the physical and mental tasks required for selected field of work or endeavor. *Personal Self* – Ideals are not firm. May have unrealistic perception of achievable goals. Sees self as a worthy being and productive.	**One is capable of developing and maintaining *mutually satisfying* autonomous and interdependent relationships with significant others and support system for one's affectional, developmental and resource adequacy needs.**
2. Prepares for selection of mate and marriage.	- Friend - Date - Roommate - Confidant	*Physical Self* – Confirms that one has ability to be a sexual partner by defining & accepting one's body image, physical characteristics & sexuality. Controls sexual urges *Personal Self* – Own sexual orientation, value system & lifestyle preference dictate type of relationship and with whom it is developed. Tend to choose individuals with similar tastes & interests or characteristics that are acceptable in a friend or potential mate.	One is able to commit oneself to an exclusive relationship for life, adjusting to a heterosexual or to a variant companionship through autonomous interdependent friendship.

(cont'd next page)

3. Refines a value system and/or code of ethics and develops socially responsible behavior.	Member of interest group, church or religious group, political party or community actions group, voter, neighbor.	*Physical Self* – Sees self as fully mature adult capable of taking on duties and responsibilities of social group.	
4. Develops a civic consciousness.	Member of social, political, religious or community action group; member of the military, political party. Voter, concerned citizen, patron; consumer advocate, etc.	*Personal Self* – Sees and tries to confirm own Self Ideal and Moral/Ethical value systems – may question or rebel against controls or restrictions imposed by family, government or institution. Compares reality with own ideals in relation to self and one may modify own ideals and value systems. Feedback from others influences values and behaviors.	
YOUNG ADULTS IN THE FAMILY ESTABLISHMENT PHASE: (25-35 yrs.) 1. Primary task is to be able to nurture, support & provide for one's mate and offspring. - Housing arrangements for family - Meeting financial needs for family - Maintaining satisfactory marriage	- Wage earner - Husband - Wife - Mother - Father - Parent - Homemaker - Head of household	*Physical Self* – Sees oneself as potential producer of children, capable of being pregnant or fathering a child, and accepts the bodily changes *Personal Self* – Self Ideal and Moral/Ethical self influences one's view on parenting and meeting expectations of others in the care of family; family	**Adult (25-35 yrs.) in Family Establishment Phase:** Develops mutually satisfying relationship with spouse or exclusive companion. Develops relationship with offspring and getting satisfaction in nurturing.

- Working out family relationships and cultivating relationships with relatives - Working out suitable philosophy of life - Establishing ties with life in community		planning and birth control conform to one's moral-ethical beliefs. Self-consistency influences one's child-rearing practices, discipline, and whether wife/mother works outside of home.	
THE GENERATIVE ADULT: (35-65 yrs.) This period of life is characterized by stability, productivity and self actualization. 1. Maintaining established economic standard and quality of living.	- Head of household - Homeowner (renter) - Taxpayer - Homemaker - Employee (or employer)	*Physical Self* – Feels healthy and strong enough to work. *Personal Self* – Feels safe and proud that has acquired most of the material things desired. Now concerned more about the quality of life – more emphasis on intangible things, such as happiness and integrity.	*Middle scene I* – (35-50 yrs.) Enhances or redevelops intimacy with one's spouse or the permanent life partner. Develops and maintains a few deep friendships.
2. Assisting children in their growth and development.	- Parent - Role Model - Reformer - Grandparent	*Physical Self* – Has health & energy to be involved in task but also aware of aging changes in self. *Personal Self* – Confirms own values & beliefs & wants to impart them to next generation; stressing moral values; may use compensatory means if have no children of own, such as Big Sister or	*Middle Scene II* – (50-65 yrs.) Develops mutually supportive relationships with grown offspring and members of the younger generation.

(cont'd next page)

3. Develops leisure time activities.	Various secondary and tertiary roles related to types of sports, arts, music, and other interest group activities.	*Physical Self* – Sees and perceives body as athletic, skillful and having energy level for activity. *Personal Self* – Gains feeling of self satisfaction from activity. May model ideal self after a well-known person.	Brother, Scout or camp leader. Shows tolerance & understanding of others rather than stressing differences and prejudices. The leisure time activities provide opportunities to meet new friends and maintain the old relationships.
4. Relating to one's mate as a person other than a role.	- Companion - Lover - Sharer - Confidant - Partner	*Personal Self* – Is aware of personal needs to be more than just "Mom" or "Dad"; has interest in things other than those related to mate, children, and home. Feels it is important to understand & discuss national & world affairs; sees self as multidimensional rather than just one role.	*Middle Scene II* (Cont'd) (50-65 yrs.) Re-evaluates and redefines one's relationship with spouse or the permanent life partner in order to enhance the relationship; the relationship may have a new meaning.
5. Accepts and adjusts to physiological changes of late middle years.	- Primary role of stated age and sex.		*Physical Self* – Has to accept and work with some of the physical & physiological changes; adopting ways to maintain or improve own health: wrinkles, middle-age

6. Retaining relationships & assisting aging parents/in-laws.	- Daughter - Son - Son-in-law - Daughter-in-law - Niece - Nephew	spread, gray hair or loss of hair, changes in strength and stamina may change one's body image. *Self Consistency* – Has to cope, at times, with fear of being "out of condition," emergence of some chronic health condition, and the effects of hormonal changes. *Personal Self* – Sees responsibility for attention & assistance to parents. May identify with parents when own children are grown.	Role reversal may happen in the relationship with one's parents or in-laws.
THE MATURE ADULT: **(Over 65 yrs.)** The major life task for the mature adult is to achieve ego integrity and satisfaction. The retirement years are a time of enjoyment and contentment with a freedom of activity previously unknown. 1. Adjusting to decreased physical strength and declining health.	Primary role of sex and age.	*Physical Self* – Feelings and perceptions about altered body image and function due to changes of aging and health problems. May experience feelings of loss of control and memory about some events.	

2. Coping with retirement and a changed financial status. Pursuing a secondary career, new interest, hobbies and/or community activity.	- Retired worker	*Personal Self* – Seeks new ways to structure time of the day & keep self occupied; finds new value or purpose to life through activities chosen. May become more free to say & do things as one pleases.	
3. Maintaining a satisfactory living arrangement.	- Homemaker - Head of household - Renter - Guest in children's home	*Physical Self*–Sees self capable of taking care of own home or apartment; able to do own shopping, cleaning, etc. *Personal Self* – May feel more secure and less threatened having personal possessions and familiar things in room; feelings of loss if have to give up home; may need to work out feelings about alternative living arrangement in retirement or rest home.	
4. Adjusting to the death of one's spouse, and loss of significant others.	- Widow(er) - Relative - Friend	*Physical Self* – Death of spouse brings intense awareness of one's own mortality. Feels enough physical strength as well as emotional stamina to take on new or extra responsibilities.	Loss of spouse may lead to deprivation of affectional and resource adequacies.

		Personal Self – Previous experiences with loss may affect how one copes with loss of spouse & loved ones. Views of self ideal & values will determine behaviors re: remarriage, dating, etc.	Adjusting to the death of spouse and going through the Loss/Grief process; one's relationships with own children and significant others take a new importance.
5. Reworking relationship with own grown children, relatives and others.	- Parent - Grandparent - Aunt, Uncle - Friend	*Personal Self* – Sees oneself as a mature adult, responsible for own health & other life affairs. Is able to make own decisions, but takes opinions of others, particularly own children. Would like to be a worthwhile contributor to the family and society with different things to offer.	
6. Assuming a new pattern of social & civic responsibilities.	Members of church or religious affiliation, political party, interest group, retirement organization, etc.	*Physical Self* – Sees self as healthy and in control of one's own body and mind for the activities. Changes in health and body image may restrict the activities. *Personal Self* – Chooses activities and interactions with people who have a value system similar to one's own. Continues feeling useful and proud to be a contributing member of society.	Membership in and contribution to social and civic organizations may, in return, provide a means of developing and maintaining network of support system for self.

Introduction to Assessment of the Self Concept Mode

According to the Roy's Adaptation Model, Self Concept is defined as the composite of image, beliefs and feelings that a person holds about one's self at a given time. The underlying basic need is one's **psychic integrity** – the need to know who one is so that one can exist with a sense of unity. It is one's own total appraisal of oneself: physical appearance and sensations, abilities to deal with life situation, future aspirations, and moral/ethical and spiritual views.

One's self concept plays a very important role in almost every moment of a person's daily living. It works as a dynamic force underlying one's behavior in a given time. Virtually every aspect of an adult's life in a given time is affected by one's self concept: where one is, what one is doing, and how one is doing.

Self concept serves as mediator between our external world and our internal world. It affects all four modes of adaptation. When and if one sees one's self as one who meets the expectations set by self as well as by others, there will be harmony, and psychic integrity will be maintained. In this case, the individual is said to have a positive self concept. The individuals with positive self concepts tend to cope with everyday adaptation problems better than those who have negative self concepts.

Presented on the following page are some of the sample summaries of the 1st level assessment of self concept mode along with a list of common nursing diagnoses in self concept mode. The student is, for practice, to match each summary of behaviors with an appropriate nursing diagnosis.

Behavioral Manifestations	Possible Nursing Diagnoses
A. Expresses change(s)/dissatisfaction in bodily appearance or functions, and demonstrates difficulties in accepting and adjusting to the new self.	• Positive Self Concept • Body image disturbance

B. Expresses or demonstrates Loss/ Grief over loss of body part(s) or function, or personal loss of valued source of psychological gratification such as loved ones, relationships, social status or things.	• _____ stage of Loss/Grieving process over:
	  - Loss of body part(s) or function
	  - Personal loss of _____

C. Expresses feelings of being unable to measure up to one's usual self and demonstrates anxiety.	• Feelings of Inadequacy or Anxiety

D. Expresses feelings of not being in control of own personal affairs or demonstrates anger and frustration, or insecurity, helplessness and hopelessness.	• Feelings of Powerlessness
	  - Physical loss of control
	  - Psychological loss of control

E. Expresses or demonstrates the feelings that one's own actions or thoughts are not in terms with the Moral, Ethical or Spiritual standards set according to one's own beliefs and value systems.	• Feelings of guilt • Low Self Esteem
F. Expresses negative outlook for life in general with feelings of discouragement, isolation, and self worthlessness. Not able to defend self, fearful of self exposure and angering others, and expects not to be accepted by others.	
G. Expresses positive outlook for life in general. Perceives and accepts oneself as one is, with intention of improving any self deficits that are within one's power to change, not focusing on those that are not.	

Assessment of Self Concept Mode

1st Level Assessment		2nd Level Assessment	Possible Nursing Diagnoses
COMPONENTS	BEHAVIORS		

A. Physical Self: *Body Sensation* How one's own body feels to oneself: "I feel _____." *Body Image* Body traits: How one's own body looks to oneself including likes and dislikes of the appearance and the functions. "I must look like _____." **B. Personal Self:** *Self Consistency* The stabilizing/organizing forces of self – usual personality traits; the kind of person one thinks one is usually in relation to actual performance or response to various situations. "I am usually _____ person."	**A. Physical Self:** 1. How does the person feel physically now in terms of his bodily functions and health? 2. What kind of body image does the person have? 3. How satisfied is the person with own physical health and body image? 4. Is person experiencing feelings of "Loss/Grief" due to change in body image or health? **B. Personal Self:** 1. What kind of person does he/she think he/she is in terms of personal characteristics? *Usual* capability; strong points as well as weak points. 2. Does the person feel he/she is measuring up to usual self? 3. Is the person experiencing any feelings of inadequacy or	**I. Age:** Growth and developmental norms expected of the person and how well the person is meeting them. **II. Responses from others:** (Interaction with others) What kind of appraisal is the person receiving from others? **III. Perception:** Is the person able to exercise cognitive function? **IV. Present Physical, Mental, & Psychosocial capabilities:** How effectively is the person managing the events happening to self and others? **V. Number and severity of current stressors and challenges one is faced with at the present time:**	Potential or Actual
			- Positive Self Concept
			- Loss and grief over changes in:
			  Physical Self – Body Image Disturbance
			  Personal Self – Loss of significant others, relationships, social status, or things that are a valued source of psychological gratification to oneself
			- Feelings of inadequacy or anxiety
			- Feelings of powerlessness; feelings of loss of control:
			  Physical
			  Psychological
			- Feelings of guilt
			- Low self-esteem

Self-Ideal/Self-Expectancy

The striving force of self – the kind of person one desires to be in terms of personal capability, aspirations, and future goals.

"I would like to be _____."

"I want to _____."

"I will _____."

Moral-Ethical-Spiritual Self

The standard setter of self – one's moral/ethical and spiritual views of self; one's beliefs and value system with the sense of rightness and wrongness.

"I believe in _____."

"I should _____."

"I should not _____."

---

anxiety due to perception of threats to self consistency?

1. What are some self expectations in terms of personal goals & aspirations, for immediate or long term future?

2. Does the person feel the expectations and personal goals are achievable and hopeful to accomplish them?

3. Is the person experiencing a feeling of powerlessness because he/she thinks he/she will not be able to meet the expectations?

1. What are some of the strong beliefs & values held by the person in terms of moral/ethical standards & spiritual need?

2. Does the person feel he/she is measuring up to the standard and acting according to the beliefs and values?

3. Is the person experiencing a feeling of guilt because he/she is not acting according to the beliefs and values?

- Disease and illness
- Surgery which may have resulted in loss of bodily function or body part(s)
- Personal losses of any kind – person, relationships, social status or things that are the person's valued source of psychological gratification

VI. Resources available for coping with stressors:
- Financial
- Personal assistance and support

VII. Other:
- Learning – past experiences with successes or failures
- cultural values and beliefs of the society and one's own

Introduction to Assessment of Role Function Mode

A role is the functioning unit of society. The society creates and deletes positions as needed for its people to carry out the role functions in order to maintain itself, protect its members, pass on its culture, and provide the most satisfying life for its members. Each role comes with a set of expectations as to how the person playing out the role function should behave toward a person playing the reciprocal role. Those expectations are the socio-cultural norms of the society and learned through socialization, observations, experiences, and formal/informal education. **Therefore, the assessment of a role function requires setting a criteria according to the socio-cultural expectations of the role function, and the person's actual role behaviors are to be compared to the set criteria for a judgment.**

Throughout one's life, a person acquires and relinquishes many roles according to the stage of life one is stationed in and other life circumstances: **Is the person occupying appropriate roles for his/her developmental stage? And, how well is the person performing according to the set of expectations?** The person's social integrity is considered to be the underlying basic need – the need to know who one is in relation to others so that one can act appropriately.

Through adaptation in role function mode, one fulfills one's social obligations to others and society. One's self actualization is also accomplished through role function mode. Further more, the kinds of roles one occupies and how well he/she plays out the roles affects the person's self concept and satisfaction in life.

Presented on the following page are the sample summaries of the 1st level assessment in role function mode along with a list of possible nursing diagnoses. The student is, for practice, to match each summary with an appropriate nursing diagnosis.

Manifesting Behaviors	Possible Nursing Diagnoses
A. The role behaviors meet the set of expectations set by the society in both Instrumental as well as Expressive components.	• Role Mastery
B. The role behaviors demonstrate adaptive Expressive behaviors with a few adaptive Instrumental behaviors that meet social expectations.	• Effective Role Transition • Ineffective Role Transition
C. The performance behaviors demonstrate both Instrumental and Expressive behaviors that meet the expectations; however, they are significantly different and at a minimum level because the role is incompatible with one's self concept.	• Role Distance • Intra-role Conflict • Inter-role Conflict • Role Failure
D. The role behaviors fail to demonstrate either appropriate Instrumental or Expressive behaviors, or both, as a result of having more than one set of expectations that are incompatible.	
E. The role behaviors fail to demonstrate either appropriate Instrumental or Expressive behaviors as a result of occupying two or more incompatible roles.	
F. The role behaviors demonstrate adaptive Expressive behaviors but exhibit ineffective Instrumental behaviors due to lack of knowledge, education, or the absence of a role model.	
G. There is an absence of Expressive and/or Instrumental role behaviors. Or, demonstration of ineffective Expressive and Instrumental behaviors.	

Assessment of Role Function Mode

1st Level Assessment		2nd Level Assessment	Possible Nursing Diagnoses
Assessment Parameter:* Identify the particular role function you are to assess and *list the expected adaptive behaviors* according to the components.	**Assess the person's *actual* *behaviors*** through observation, interview and requiring the client to demonstrate, if necessary, and compare them to the expected adaptive behaviors.	Review all the stimuli affecting one's role behaviors in order to identify the particular stimuli causing ineffective behaviors.	**Nursing Diagnosis:** See which of the following is applicable to the assessed behaviors and stimuli.
Instrumental (expected)	*Instrumental (actual)*	**I. Presence or absence of the 4 partitions of role function:**	Potential or Actual
		- Consumer/Beneficiary	- **Role Mastery**
		- Access to Facility/Set of Circumstances	- **Effective Role Transition**
		- Cooperation/Collaboration from Others	
		- Remuneration/Reward	- **Ineffective Role Transition**
		II. Cultural orientation or familiarity to the required role performance behaviors	- **Role Distance**
			- **Inter-role Conflict**
		III. Required vs. actual physical, mental and emotional capabilities, and appropriateness of developmental stage of the person for the role	- **Intra-role Conflict**
			- **Role Failure**

Expressive (expected)	Expressive (actual)
	IV. Self concept of the role performer
	V. Acceptance of the role behaviors by the person playing the reciprocating role(s)
	VI. Adequacy of knowledge and practice
	VII. Availability of role model
	VIII. Other: - Number and type of roles one is assuming and how compatible they are with each other - Different/conflicting role expectations from others

*Setting criteria for judgment is needed in order to evaluate the person's actual role performance behaviors. They are the written or unwritten social expectations; the expected role behaviors of a 4th grade student would be different from that of a college student.

18

Assessment of Interdependence Mode

Interdependence Mode is one of the three psychosocial adaptation modes in the Roy Adaptation Model. It focuses on the close relationships of people, their purpose, structure and development.

The underlying basic need is the **relational integrity** which is related to meeting one's need for affection, progression through normal development, and resources needed for healthy living. In order to meet these needs, a person has to develop and maintain interdependent relationships through effective interactions with others.

An Interdependent relationship is characterized by a willingness and ability to give to and accept from others whatever one can offer: love, respect, value, nurturing, time, commitment, material possessions, and knowledge. Though the balance between the giving and accepting changes through different stages of one's life, it is through such relationships that one continues to grow as an individual and as a healthy contributing member of society.

Therefore, next to the biological integrity, relational integrity is considered the most important basic need for one's survival and overall adaptation in life.

Assessment of the Interdependence Mode focuses on **how well the person's needs for Affectional adequacy, Developmental adequacy, and Resource adequacy are met.**

Presented on the following page are the sample summaries of the 1st level assessment along with a list of the possible diagnoses. The student is, for practice, to match each summary with an appropriate nursing diagnosis.

Manifesting Behaviors	Possible Nursing Diagnoses
A. Is not able to name any significant others or support system	• Ineffective Pattern of Giving and Receiving
B. Does not effectively interact with others: Does not express love/affection, respect, and value to others in such a way they can recognize and appreciate. Does not assimilate (respond to) the love, affection, respect, and value expressed by others in such a way that it encourages the others to continue.	• Ineffective Pattern of Dependency and Independency • Separation Anxiety • Inability to Develop or Maintain Interdependent Relationships: Loneliness • Inadequate Network of Significant Others and Support System
C. Is separated physically from the significant others and support system.	• Inadequate Resources
D. Demonstrates inappropriate dependent and independent behaviors for the person's developmental stage.	
F. Person's basic food, shelter, and clothing needs are not being adequately met.	
G. Is not able or does not know how to initiate contact with others to develop and maintain close relationships.	

Assessment of Interdependence Mode

1st Level Assessment	2nd Level Assessment of Stimuli-Influencing Factor	Possible Nursing Diagnoses
Affectional Adequacy:	**Affectional Adequacy:**	Actual or potential
I. Structural Components:	I. Self-awareness of need for affectional adequacy	- Inadequate network of significant others and support system
Does the person maintain an adequate network of significant others/support system, & maintain good relationships with them?	II. Expectation of the relationship	- Ineffective pattern of giving and receiving
A. Significant others:	III. Growth and developmental stage and appropriateness for the type of relationship	
- Who are the most important person(s) in your life?	IV. Actual presence/proximity of the structural components	- Separation Anxiety
- What kind of relationships do you have with significant other(s)? How satisfying are your relationships with your significant others?	V. Self-concept/Self-esteem	- Inability/ineffective development of relationships; loneliness
- Are your significant others readily available to meet your needs?	VI. Knowledge and skills required for nurturing	
B. Support system:	VII. Knowledge about human relationships and friendship	
- What support systems do you have?	VIII. Interactional skills	
- What are your expectations of them and are they meeting your expectations?		
- Are they readily available?		

2. Interactional components:
Does the person demonstrate effective Interactional Behavior?

Interpersonal:

Does the person express love, affection and respect to others in such a way they can recognize and appreciate?

Does the person assimilate or respond to the love, affection, respect, and value expressed by others in such a way that it encourages the others to continue?

A. Receptive (Receiving)
- What kind of nurturing do you receive from your significant others?
- How do you receive (assimilate) the nurturing actions demonstrated by your significant other(s)?

B. Contributive (Giving)
- In what way do you carry out your nurturing for your significant other(s)?
- How do your significant others assimilate your affection and nurturing?

C. Do you initiate/maintain contact with others for close relationships?

(cont'd next page)

IX. Receptiveness of the complementary role player

X. Availability of time and resources to develop and maintain relationships

Developmental Adequacy:

1. Is the person involved in relationships that are appropriate to his/her developmental stage? Are the relationships conducive to a healthy balance between the dependency and independency appropriate for the person's age, gender, and other physical, mental, or emotional inequities?

A. Dependency:

- Is the person able to rely on the significant other for support, attention, and affection?

- Are the behaviors of seeking support, attention, and affection appropriate for developmental stage?

B. Independency:

- Does the person take initiative for independent actions for oneself?

- Are the behaviors of taking initiative for independent actions appropriate for the person's developmental stage ?

Resource Adequacy:

1. Are the person's basic physical needs adequately met? Are the significant others and support system contributing in meeting the needs?

- food   - shelter   - clothing

Developmental Adequacy:

I. The person's developmental stage

II. Physical, mental, or emotional conditions

III. Having personal crisis

IV. The person's self concept

V. Knowledge about friendship and how to maintain

Resource Adequacy:

I. Availability of financial resources

II. Availability of assistance

- Ineffective pattern of dependency and independency

- Inadequate resource

98

Self Critiquing of Nursing Care Plan

1. **The 1st Level Assessment:** Assessment of Behaviors (responses to the stimuli)

   Did I assess most of the essential behaviors for the particular mode/need I am focusing on now?

   And, have I recognized the ineffective behaviors by circling them?

2. **The 2nd Level Assessment:** Assessment of stimuli (influencing factors)

   Did I assess most of the essential stimuli (Influencing Factors) that are the common causes for the behaviors in the 1st level assessment?

   And, have I recognized the particular *negative* stimuli that have caused the ineffective behaviors I have circled in the 1st level assessment?

3. **The Nursing Diagnosis:** Defining the patient's adaptation problem

   Is the diagnosis well validated by a cluster (more than one behavior) of **Manifesting ineffective behaviors** from the 1st level assessment and the specific **Stimuli** from the 2nd level assessment?

   Are the stimuli under **Due to** listed according to *Focal, Contextual* and *Residual* stimuli?

   And, do the listed ineffective behaviors and the listed stimuli reflect the **cause and effect** relationship?

4. **The Nursing Goal:** Anticipated behavioral outcome to be accomplished by the patient

   Is the Nursing Goal reflective of the Nursing Diagnosis? Does it directly deal with the problem the nursing diagnosis is presenting?

   Is the Nursing Goal stated as **the patient's behavioral outcome** (*The patient will...*) with expected time frame and criteria for evaluation?

5. **The Nursing Intervention:** The plan of actions that will be carried out by the nurse in order to assist the patient in achieving the stated nursing goal
   Will the listed nursing interventions produce the behavioral outcome stated in the nursing goal?
   Do the listed nursing interventions directly deal with the stated goal?
   Did I work with all the specific stimuli listed under the **Due to** to change, remove or reduce the negative stimuli?

6. **Evaluation/Modification:** Measurement of the outcome
   Is the Evaluation validated by the presence or lack of the desired outcome behaviors stated in the nursing goal?
   Is the Modification based on reassessment of the behaviors and stimuli?

Reference:

Roy, Sister Callista and Heather A. Andrews. *Roy Adaptation Model,* 1st and 2nd Edition. Appleton & Lange, 1999.

Four Modes of Adaptation: Common Nursing Diagnoses

Modes of Adaptation	Sub-Components	Common Adaptation Challenges: Nursing Diagnoses

Psycho Social Mode: <u>**Self Concept Mode:**</u> Maintains Psychic Integrity by meeting the need to know <u>"who am I",</u> so one can be and exist with a sense of unity.	Physical Self: - Body image - Body Sensation
	
	Body Self: - Self Consistency - Self Ideal - Moral-Ethical/ Spiritual Self
		• Body Image Disturbance
		• In _____ stage of Loss/Grieving Process is over:
		  - Loss of Body Part(s) or Function(s)
		  - Personal Loss of _____
		• Feelings of Anxiety
		• Feeling of Powerlessness over:
		  - Physical Loss of Control
		  - Psychological Loss of Control
		• Feelings of Guilt
		• Low Self-Esteem

<u>**Role Function Mode:**</u> Maintains Social integrity by meeting the need to know <u>"who am I in relation to others",</u> and acting (play the role) appropriately according to social expectations.	Roles: - Primary - Secondary - Tertiary Role Behaviors: - Instrumental - Expressive	• Role Mastery • Effective Role Transition • Ineffective Role Transition • Role Distance • Intra-Role Conflict • Inter-Role Conflict • Role Failure
<u>**Interdependence Mode:**</u> Maintains **Relational Integrity** by meeting the need to have close relationships with others.	Affectional Adequacy Developmental Adequacy Resource Adequacy	• Ineffective Pattern of Giving and Receiving • Ineffective pattern of Dependency and Independency • Inadequate Resources • Inability to Develop and Maintain Interdependent Relationships— Loneliness • Inadequate Network of Significant Others and Support System

Four Modes of Adaptation: Common Nursing Diagnoses

Modes of Adaptation	Sub-Components	Common Adaptation Challenges: Nursing Diagnoses
Physiological Mode: Maintains <u>Biological Integrity</u> by meeting the basic Physiological needs: - Oxygenation - Fluid/ Electrolyte Regulation - Nutrition - Elimination - Rest/Activity - Neurosensory Regulation - Protection	Oxygenation Need	• Inability to maintain adequate airway • Ineffective breathing pattern • Negative 02 balance: - Confusion / Disorientation - Potential for physical injury - Activity Intolerance • Hyperventilation • Hypoventilation* • Impending Shock • Potential for Medical Complication in cardio / Vascular / Pulmonary System* • Self Care Knowledge deficit
	Fluid & Electrolytes Regulation Need	• Dehydration: - Early Stage or Advanced Stage • Electrolyte Imbalance;* - Hypo - Hyper • Fluid Overload:* - Early stage or Advanced Stage • Self Care Knowledge Deficit
	Nutritional Need	• Inadequate Caloric Intake • Excessive Caloric Intake • Nutritional Deficiency in _____ (specific elements) • Altered Means of Nutritional Intake • Self-Care Knowledge Deficit
	Solid Elimination Need	• Discomfort of Flatulence • Inadequate Bowel Elimination - Constipation - Fecal Impaction • Problems associated with Excessive Bowel Elimination - Discomfort - Loss of body F/E and Nutritional Element - Cross Contamination • Altered Means of Solid Elimination • Self Care Knowledge Deficit

Four Modes of Adaptation: Common Nursing Diagnoses

Modes of Adaptation	Sub-Components	Common Adaptation Challenges: Nursing Diagnoses

Physiological Mode continued:	Fluid Elimination Need	• Loss of Urinary Control:*
		  - Urinary Incontinence
		  - Urinary Retention
		• Potential for Urinary Tract Infection
		• Dysuria Secondary to Urinary Tract Infection
		• Altered Means of Fluid Elimination
		• Self Care Knowledge Deficit

	Rest / Activity Need	• Inadequate Physical Activity / Potential for Development of Disuse Syndrome • Activity Intolerance / Potential for Physical Injury • Disuse Syndrome • REM Sleep Deprivation • Total Sleep Deprivation • Insomnia • Self Care Knowledge Deficit

	Neurosensory Regulation Need	• Problems associated with known Neuro-Sensory Deficit:
		  - Confusion / Disorientation
		  - Potential for Physical Injury
		  - Inability to carry out ADL
		  - Difficulty in Communication
		  - Learning to Live with Neuro-Sensory Limitations
		• Sensory-Perceptual Deprivation
		• Sensory-Perceptual Overload
		• Pain
		• Discomfort—Aberrant Sensation

	Protection Need	• Inability to Maintain Physical Safety
		• Effects of Impaired Skin Integrity
		  - Secondary Infection
		  - Loss of Body Fluid
		  - Discomfort or Pain

		*-Need collaboration with Medical Intervention